Dysfunctional Uterine Bleeding

Advances in
Reproductive
Endocrinology

VOLUME 2

Dysfunctional Uterine Bleeding

Edited by RW Shaw

The Parthenon Publishing Group
International Publishers in Science, Technology & Education

Casterton Hall, Carnforth,
Lancs, LA6 2LA, UK

120 Mill Road, Park Ridge,
New Jersey, USA

Published in the UK by
The Parthenon Publishing Group Limited
Casterton Hall, Carnforth,
Lancs, LA6 2LA, England

Published in the USA by
The Parthenon Publishing Group Inc.
120 Mill Road,
Park Ridge,
New Jersey 07656, USA

Copyright © Parthenon Publishing Group Ltd

British Library Catologuing in Publication Data
Dysfunctional uterine bleeding.
  1. Women. Menstruation. Disorders. Role of endocrine system
  I.   Shaw, Robert W. (Robert Wayne)   II. Series
  618.172071

  ISBN 1-85070-296-9
  ISBN 0-929858-49-2 U.S.

Library of Congress Cataloging-in-Publication Data
  Dysfunctional uterine bleeding / edited by R.W. Shaw.
       p.   cm. - - (Advances in reproductive endocrine research)
     Contains proceedings from the First Symposia in Reproductive Endocrine
  Disorders, held at St. John's College, Cambridge in September 1989.
     Includes bibliographical references.
     ISBN 0-929858-49-2 : $45.00
     1. Hemorrhage, Uterine - - Congresses.   2. Hemorrhage, Uterine - -
  Chemotherapy - - Congresses.   I. Shaw, Robert W. (Robert Wayne)
  II. Symposia in Reproductive Endocrine Disorders (1st : 1989 : Cambridge,
  England) III. Series.
     [DNLM: 1. Uterine Hemorrhage - - physiopathology - -
  congresses.   WP 400 D9983 1989]
  RG711.D96   1990
  618.1'72 - - dc20
  DNLM/DLC
  for Library of Congress   90-8920
                                                                        CIP

First published 1990

Composition by Ryburn Typesetting Ltd, Halifax, England
Printed and bound in Great Britain by
Butler and Tanner, Frome and London

Contents

List of principal contributors   vii

Foreword   ix

1.   Physiology of normal menstruation   1
     S.K. Smith

2.   Prostaglandin dysfunction in dysfunctional uterine bleeding   13
     M.C.P. Rees

3.   Coagulation and electron microscopy studies in menorrhagia   25
     B.L. Sheppard

4.   Phospholipases – a role in dysfunctional uterine bleeding?   43
     R.C. Bonney, J. Higham, J.S. Beesley, H. Watson and S. Franks

5.   Evaluation of menstrual blood loss – value of history and   59
     subjective assessment
     M.P. Lamb

6.   Measured menstrual blood losses – normal population and   69
     'menorrhagic' patients
     J.M. Higham and R.W. Shaw

7.   Menorrhagia – the cost and scope of treatment   85
     M.A. Lumsden

8. Endometrial ablation techniques   97
    A.L. Magos

9. The use of prostaglandin synthetase inhibitors in dysfunctional   117
    uterine bleeding
    C.J. Dockeray

10. Danazol in dysfunctional uterine bleeding   127
    R.W. Shaw

11. Treatment of dysfunctional uterine bleeding with oral,   139
    intramuscular or intrauterine progestogens
    I.S. Fraser

12. LHRH analogues in the treatment of menorrhagia   149
    R. Gardner and R.W. Shaw

    Index   161

List of principal contributors

R.C. Bonney
Department of Chemical
  Pathology
St Mary's Hospital Medical School
London W2 1PG
UK

C.J. Dockeray
Charlemont Clinic
Charlemont Mall
Dublin 2
Eire

I.S. Fraser
Department of Obstetrics and
  Gynaecology
University of Sydney
NSW 2006
Australia

R. Gardner
Academic Department of
  Obstetrics and Gynaecology
Royal Free Hospital
Pond Street
London NW3 2QG
UK

J.M. Higham
Academic Department of
  Obstetrics and Gynaecology
Royal Free Hospital
Pond Street
London NW3 2QG
UK

M.P. Lamb
County Hospital
Greetwell Road
Lincoln LN2 5QY
UK

M.A. Lumsden
Department of Obstetrics and
    Gynaecology
Western General Hospital
Crewe Road
Edinburgh EH4 2XU
UK

A.L.Magos
Nuffield Department of
    Obstetrics and Gynaecology
University of Oxford
John Radcliffe Hospital
Maternity Department
Oxford OX3 9DU
UK

M.C.P. Rees
Nuffield Department of
    Obstetrics and Gynaecology
University of Oxford
John Radcliffe Hospital
Maternity Department
Oxford OX3 9DU
UK

R.W. Shaw
Academic Department of
    Obstetrics and Gynaecology
Royal Free Hospital
Pond Street
London NW3 2QG
UK

B.L. Sheppard
Trinity College Department of
    Obstetrics and Gynaecology
Sir Patrick Dun Research Centre
St James's Hospital
Dublin 8
Eire

S.K. Smith
Department of Obstetrics and
    Gynaecology
University of Cambridge
Rosie Maternity Hospital
Robinson Way
Cambridge CB2 2SW
UK

Foreword

The problem of dysfunctional uterine bleeding – excessive or prolonged regular menstrual bleeding in the absence of overt uterine pathology, endocrine or haematological disorder – is a common reason for General Practitioner consultation and a significant proportion of referrals to Gynaecological Out-patient Departments. In recent years basic physiological research has resulted in a greater depth of insight into the mechanisms involved in the control of normal menstruation and the pathophysiology of dysfunctional uterine bleeding. Newer drug therapies and the development of less invasive surgical techniques mean that this area of clinical gynaecological practice is in need of an in-depth review. These proceedings, resulting from our second workshop in Reproductive Endocrinology, held at St. John's College, Cambridge in September 1989 [and kindly sponsored by ICI Pharmaceuticals], have aimed to do just that.

The first four chapters evaluate the physiological mechanisms involved in control of menstruation and menstrual blood loss endeavouring to define the role of disordered prostaglandin synthesis, alteration in phospholipase A_2 production and platelet and coagulation factors. The inter-relation of these factors and the newer evidence accruing on the role of growth factors and regeneration of the endometrium indicate that the story is as yet far from resolved.

The necessity to evaluate blood loss in patients presenting with menorrhagia carefully and objectively is clear from the data presented in Chapters 5 and 6, where all current clinical evaluations utilized in normal history taking are questioned. Whilst accurate objective blood loss measurements using alkaline haematin dilution techniques are accurate they are unlikely to be used on a wide scale in clinical practice. The development of other means of assessment is essential and the Pictorial Blood Loss Assessment Chart (PBAC) looks to be an exciting development.

The enormous scope and cost of the disorder is reviewed in Chapter 7 whilst Chapter 8 investigates the potential for endometrial ablation techniques, a new change in surgical approach which needs careful and full evaluation.

Finally in the remaining chapters the current medical treatments utilizing prostaglandin synthetase inhibitors, danazol, progestogens and gonadotropin-releasing hormone analogues are reviewed in depth and evaluated.

These proceedings provide a comprehensive and up-to-date in depth review of the topic of dysfunctional uterine bleeding and should provide relevant data for every gynaecologist.

Academic Department of Obstetrics
   and Gynaecology
Royal Free Hospital
London NW3 2QG, UK

Professor Robert W. Shaw
November 1989

1

Physiology of normal menstruation

S.K. Smith

MENSTRUAL FUNCTION

Menstrual dysfunction is an important cause of ill health in women. The mechanisms underlying normal menstruation remain poorly understood. The changing role of women in society as they seek employment outside of the home has increased the social problems that menstrual dysfunction eschews. Similarly, the widespread use of oral contraception and now hormone replacement therapy, with their important side-effects of breakthrough bleeding and withdrawal bleeds, has raised important questions about the factors which regulate menstrual bleeding in women. In this chapter I will concentrate on the mechanisms already known to be involved in the process of menstruation and will speculate on some of the areas where new discoveries may shed light on to this complicated mechanism.

The endocrine basis of menstruation

In a normal cycle the regression of the corpus luteum is associated with declining levels of oestradiol and progesterone. Withdrawal of oestradiol and progesterone from a previously primed endometrium will always result in menstrual bleeding in women. It appears that the most important component of the declining steroid levels is the withdrawal of progesterone, as although bleeding may occur on some occasions with withdrawal of oestradiol, maintained levels of progesterone will prevent withdrawal bleeding. However, a consequence of maintained levels of progesterone is a high frequency (between 15 and 25%) of breakthrough bleeding which does not appear to be associated with altered levels of peripheral steroid. Thus, at least two mechanisms appear to exist in menstrual bleeding. Firstly, bleeding associated with declining levels of peripheral steroid and bleeding associated with steady state levels of peripheral steroid. Recent evidence suggests that the majority of women who present to the gynaecological clinic with a complaint of menorrhagia have regular ovulatory menstrual cycles[1]. Furthermore, daily measurements of oestradiol and progesterone in women with and without heavy periods have failed to demonstrate any significant differences in peripheral hormone levels[2]. Approximately 20% of women who present with menstrual dysfunction will have anovulatory cycles due to a series of conditions which are not appropriate to this chapter.

In the absence of obvious endocrine pathology, the need to understand basic local mechanisms of menstruation are paramount. Four basic theories have been propounded to explain the mechanism of menstruation:
(1)   Changes in vascular tone of the spiral arterioles;
(2)   Changes in the mechanisms of haemostasis in the uterus;
(3)   Alterations in lysosomal function; and
(4)   Regeneration of endometrium.

Vascular changes

The seminal work of Markee[3], in which rabbit endometrium was transplanted into the anterior chamber of the eye of the Rhesus monkey, demonstrated that menstruation was preceded by intense vasoconstriction of the spiral arterioles. This was consequent upon regression of the endometrium and an increased coiling of the spiral arteriole. This coiling was assumed to induce ischaemia but the intense vasoconstriction was a secondary phenomenon which arose from the coiling. Further evidence using hydrodynamic principles suggests that the coiling mechanism is probably not important in altering vascular flow but the intense vasoconstriction which precedes menstruation is still considered to be the important event at the start of menstruation. Once the vasoconstriction has occurred, there will be distal ischaemia and when the spiral arteriole vasodilates between 4 and 24 h after the onset of the contraction, blood passes into the ischaemic endometrium and presumably by a mechanism involving the release of free oxygen radicals, produces desquamation of the tissue. The control of menstrual bleeding then appears to rely on three mechanisms, of which one appears to be the return of vasoconstriction to the stump of the spiral arteriole. It is not known what is the agent which induces the vasoconstriction, nor is it known whether the continued vasoconstriction is responsible for the control of the blood loss, or whether other factors like platelet fibrin plug formation or angiogenic stimulus to vascular regeneration are involved in the subsequent control of menstrual bleeding.

Haemostasis

Platelet fibrin plug formation is grossly deficient in endometrium and is thus unlike clotting mechanisms in other parts of the body[4]. Ruptured spiral aterioles do form platelet fibrin thrombi in the early phases of menstruation but these are retained within the vessel and do not form the characteristic mushroom-shaped plug found in other tissues. However, by the end of the 24th hour of menstrual bleeding, the endometrium is principally devoid of this plug formation. It is not known whether platelets degranulate and coagulate in the process of passage throughout the myometrium or endometrium, or whether this occurs within the uterine cavity. However, menstrual fluid contains serum, low numbers of platelets and minimal fibrinogen, and is analogous to a post-coagulant serum[5]. The rapid formation of fibrin plugs and their degradation may play a part in the control of menstrual bleeding, and the relevant times of formation and subsequent disaggregation may be important in regulating the flow of blood into the uterine cavity.

Lysosomes

Henzl *et al.*[6] demonstrated changes in lysosomal content of endometrial cells throughout the cycle, and further experiments on liver lysosomes have demonstrated changes in the 'leakiness' of lysosomes under the influence of ovarian steroids with increased leakiness occurring with the withdrawal of progesterone. Lysosomes are assumed to contain a series of enzymes of which some of those involved with prostaglandin synthesis are maintained, and the suggestion has been that there is increased release of these enzymes on progesterone withdrawal. There is no objective evidence to substantiate this claim.

Regeneration

The endometrium undergoes regeneration almost from the beginning of menstruation, and although by the end of 24 h the outer two-thirds of the functional layer of the endometrium has been lost, the basal layer of the endometrium consists of tufts of epithelial cells extruding up from the basal glands, and a raw surface consisting of endothelial and mesenchymal cells of the stroma[7]. By the fifth day of menstruation in most cases this endometrium has undergone profound regeneration, with outgrowth of epithelial cells from the glandular tufts, and presumably significant structural reorganization of the stromal cells underlying the epithelium. Similarly, profound angiogenesis occurs at this time with repair of ruptured arterioles, veins and capillaries. It is not known to what degree the rapidity of regeneration is involved in the control of menstrual loss.

PROSTAGLANDINS AND MENSTRUATION

Introduction

Thus far the agent thought to be most likely to be involved in the vascular control of the spiral arterioles is prostaglandin. The evidence for this is that prostaglandins when instilled into the uterine cavity of the non-pregnant women, induce menstrual bleeding[8], prostaglandin synthesis inhibitors reduce menstrual blood loss[9], and prostaglandins exert vasoconstricting and vasodilating properties in a wide range of species and vascular beds which would be consistent with their role in menstruation.

Prostaglandin synthesis

Prostaglandins are released from free arachidonic acid, itself the product of phospholipase A_2 and phospholipase C activity on phosphoglycerides in the cell membrane. The rate limiting step in the synthesis of prostaglandins is the availability of free cytosolic arachidonic acid, which constitutes less than 5% of cellular arachidonic acid[10]. Prostaglandin synthetase, a group of enzymes, is then responsible for the conversion of the arachidonic acid to primary prostaglandin. The eicosanoid cascade arising from the release of free arachidonic acid also includes the lipoxygenase products, i.e. leukotrienes. The regulation of this complicated inter-related second messenger system is exceedingly complex but involves the regulation of expression of the enzymes, the structural changes of the proteins, the binding of the proteins to cell membrane, and the availability of cytosolic calcium arising from intracellular calcium pools, and from extracellular sources. Oestradiol is known to stimulate prostaglandin production[11], an effect antagonized by progesterone[12]. Furthermore, withdrawal of progesterone as determined by the effect of antiprogestins on progesterone-dominated endometria, results in increased prostaglandin synthesis[13]. Thus, the mechanism exists for steroids to prime the uterus and then, on the withdrawal of progesterone, to result in the actual enhanced synthesis of prostaglandins. Regrettably, there is little evidence to demonstrate that prostaglandin $F_{2\alpha}$ is the vasoconstricting agent responsible for the onset of menstruation, and it may be that other vasoactive substances are more potent than prostaglandins and that prostaglandins simply function in a modulatory role. However, this is not the only role that prostaglandins have to play in menstruation as they also have important effects in haemostasis and regeneration.

Prostaglandins and endometrial function

Prostaglandins also have an important part to play in the mechanism of haemostasis. Prostacyclin is one of the most potent anticoagulators yet known to man, and yet thromboxane, (derived from platelets) is integrally involved in the mechanism of platelet activation. Changes in the ratio of prostacyclin to thromboxane have been demonstrated in women with menorrhagia[14], suggesting that elevated amounts of prostacyclin results in reduced formation of platelet fibrin plugs.

The source of prostacyclins and thromboxanes in endometrium is unknown but it is likely that prostacyclin is derived from endothelial cells and that the thromboxanes are released by activated platelets. It is not clear if the altered ratio arises from an enhanced synthesis of prostacyclin or a reduced release of thromboxanes from the platelets. However, women with platelet disorders including thrombocytopenia, and von Willebrand disease, have increased menstrual blood loss[15], suggesting that platelet dysfunction may cause menorrhagia. The source of the prostaglandins in this mechanism is unknown but presumably thromboxanes are principally released from platelets, and suggests that disorders of the paracrine relationship between endometrial epithelial cells and the circulating platelets are relevant to menstrual dysfunction.

Endometrial regeneration

Thus far, attention has focused on the roles of vascular tonicity and haemostasis in the control of menstrual blood loss. However, the process of growth and differentiation in the endometrium at the time of bleeding would seem to be an important part of the control of menstrual loss with the repair of blood vessels and the repair of the tissue. Little is known of the factors which regulate endometrial proliferation, although for a long time oestradiol has been considered to be the prime mitogen. There is little evidence *in vitro* to confirm oestrogen as a mitogen in either breast or endometrial epithelial cells, and the possibility exists that it might exert its mitogenic effect by other mechanisms than by simply directly binding to its own response element in stimulating the proliferation of cells. There is considerable evidence to show that oestrogen stimulates the synthesis and/or release of polypeptide growth factors and their receptors.

Epidermal growth factor (EGF) is a 53 amino acid peptide derived from a large 1168 amino acid precursor[16,17]. Mouse endometrium has been shown to contain a 4.7 kb pre-pro-EGF message and the peptide is present on the surface of glandular and luminal epithelial cells[18]. Provisional results using the reverse transcriptase–polymerase chain reaction demonstrate that small amounts of human endometrium contains the message for mature EGF.

EGF acts by binding to a specific 170 kD, glycosylated transmembrane receptor[19]. EGF receptors are present in human endometrium[20] and in the rat, oestradiol stimulated increase in mRNA for the receptor[21]. Taken together these findings suggest that the polypeptide growth factor, EGF, may be involved in endometrial proliferation. Much work is required in elaborating this role and determining its potential effect in pathological states like menorrhagia.

EGF is not the only growth factor present in endometrium and transforming growth factors α and β have been demonstrated in endometrium (personal communication). Similarly, colony–stimulating factor 1 has been demonstrated in mouse endometrium and has been shown to stimulate proliferation of transformed human endometrial carcinoma cells[22]. There are a large number of factors which may be involved in regulating the normal proliferation of endometrial cells and recent evidence in the rabbit suggests that prostaglandins may be involved in this mechanism. This interaction of prostaglandins and growth factors in endometrial function raises the prospect of a complicated but integrated mechanism involving the ovarian steroids in the regulation of endometrial growth, by factors which could have effects on vascular tonicity, haemostasis, endometrial regeneration and angiogenesis. It is likely that research into the mechanism of menstruation in the ensuing years will be to follow these approaches.

REFERENCES

1. Cameron, I.T. (1989). Dysfunctional uterine bleeding, *Bailliere's Clin. Obstet. Gynaecol.*, **3**, 315–26
2. Haynes, P.J., Anderson, A.B.M. and Turnbull, A. (1979). Patterns of menstrual blood loss in menorrhagia. *Res. Clin. Forums*, **1**, 73–8
3. Markee, J.E. (1940). Menstruation in intraocular endometrial transplants in the rhesus monkey. *Contr. Embryol. Carnegie Inst.*, **28**, 219–308
4. Christiaens, G.C.M.L., Sixma, J.J. and Haspels, A.A. (1980). Morphology of haemastasis in menstrual endometrium. *Br. J. Obstet. Gynaecol.*, **87**, 425–39
5. Hahn, L., Cederblad, G., Rybo, G., Pehrson, G. and Kosanbentsen, K. (1976). Blood coagulation fibronolysis and plasma proteins in women with normal and excessive blood loss. *Br. J. Obstet. Gynaecol.*, **83**, 974–80
6. Henzl, M.R., Smith, R.E., Boost, G. and Tyler, E.T. (1972). Lysosomal

concept of menstrual bleeding in humans. *J. Clin. Endocrinol. Metab.*, **34**, 860–75

7. Ludwig, H. and Metzger, H. (1970). The re-epithelialization of endometrium after menstrual desquamation. *Archiv Gynekol.*, **221**, 51–60

8. Toppozada, M., El-Attar, A., El-Ayatt, M.A. and Khamis, Y. (1980). Management of uterine bleeding by PGs or their synthesis inhibition. *Adv. Prost. Thromb. Res.*, **8**, 459–63

9. Dockeray, C.J. (1988). The medical treatment of menorrhagia. In Chamberlain, G. (ed.). *Contemporary Obstetrics and Gynaecology*, pp. 229–314. (London: Butterworths)

10. Lapetina, E.G. (1982). Regulation of arachidonic acid production: role of phospholipase C and A2. *Trends Pharmacol. Sci.*, **3**, 115–18

11. Smith, S.K. and Kelly, R.W. (1988). Prostaglandin- and steroid-induced endometrial changes in early human pregnancy. *J. Reprod. Fert.*, Suppl. 36, 143–54

12. Kelly, R.W. and Smith, S.K. (1987). Progesterone and antiprogestins, a comparison of their effect on prostaglandin: production by human secretory phase endometrium and decidua. *Prost. Leuk. Med.*, **29**, 181–6

13. Smith, S.K. and Kelly, R.W. (1987). The effect of the antiprogestins RU 486 and ZK 98734 on the synthesis and metabolism of PGF2a and PGE2 in separated cells from early human decidua. *J. Clin. Endocrinol. Metab.*, **63**, 527–37

14. Makarainen, L. and Ylikorkala, O. (1986). Ibuprofen prevents IUCD-induced increases in menstrual blood loss. *Br. J. Obstet. Gynaecol.*, **93**, 285–8

15. Fraser, I.S., McCarron, G., Markham, R., Resta, T. and Watts, A. (1986). Measured menstrual blood loss in women with menorrhagia associated with pelvic disease or coagulation disorder. *Obstet. Gynecol.*, **68**, 630–3

16. Gray, A., Dull, T.J. and Ullrich, A. (1983). Nucleotide sequence of epidermal growth factor cDNA predicts a 128,000 molecular weight protein precursor. *Nature*, **303**, 722–5

17. Scott, J., Urdea, M., Quirigo, M., Sanchez-Pescador, R., Fong, N., Selby, M., Rutter, W.J. and Bell, G.I. (1983). Structure of a mouse submaxillary gland messenger RNA encoding epidermal growth factor and seven related proteins. *Science*, **221**, 236–40

18. DiAugustine, R.P., Petrusz, P., Bell, G.I., Brown, C.F., Korach, K.S., McLachlan, J.A. and Teng, C.T. (1988). Influence of estrogens on mouse uterine epidermal growth factor precursor protein and messenger ribonucleic acid. *Endocrinology*, **122**, 2355–63

19. Cohen, S., Ushiro, H., Stoscheck, C. and Chinkers, M. (1982). A native 170,000 epidermal growth factor receptor-kinase complex from shed

plasma membrane vesicles. *J. Biol. Chem.*, **257**, 1523–31

20. Hofman, G.E., Rao, C.V., Barrows, G. H., Schultz, G.S. and Sanfilippo, J.S. (1984). Binding sites for epidermal growth factor in human uterine tissues and leiomyomas. *J. Clin. Endocrinol. Metab.*, **58**, 880–4

21. Lingham, R.B., Stancel, G.M. and Loose-Mitchell, D.S. (1988). Estrogen regulation of epidermal growth factor receptor messenger ribonucleic acid. *Mol. Endocrinol.*, **2**, 230–5

22. Croxtall, J.D., Elder, M.G. and White, J.O. (1989). Steroid regulation of lipocortin II in endometrial cancer. *J. Endocrinol.*, Suppl. 121, 176–7

DISCUSSION

Prof. R.W. Shaw I was very interested in Professor Smith's suggestions on the role of the EGF and the effect that oestrogen levels may have on its function. I do not know what the time lapse is between oestrogen changes, enzyme induction and actual tissue reactivity, but he was suggesting that even by day 2 of menstruation, *in vitro* tissue is beginning to regenerate very rapidly from the gland openings. If oestrogen is the main stimulator, oestrogen levels are not changing that much between day 1 and day 2 of the cycle. Is it in fact the progesterone withdrawal that allows EGF to begin to work rather than oestrogen in itself beginning to rise?

Prof. S.K. Smith High levels of oestrogen have been used on the Continent for some years to reduce menstrual blood loss, and the actual clinical applications of oestrogen are quite well known.

It is a very complicated mechanism. For the sake of speed I stuck only to the EGF story, but it is just as likely that transforming growth factor α, which is produced from wound macrophages, is probably just as important; it binds to the same receptor. There is also colony-stimulating factor which is now known to be produced in the glandular cells of the uterus.

The fact that proliferation is important, that EGF is involved and it is influenced by steroids, begins to draw the same sort of links that we did with prostaglandins.

Mr S.M. Wood There was a hypothesis current 10 years ago that there was an importance in the difference of prostaglandin (PG)F, PGE, thromboxane and prostacyclin, but perhaps PG synthetase inhibitors might swing the balance towards the vasoconstrictor and away from vasodilator prostaglandins. Has that hypothesis now been dropped?

Prof. S.K. Smith Certainly not. We have done three separate studies in Edinburgh in which we showed differences in the ratio of prostaglandin production.

I certainly feel that the question is still very much open, that there is a change, an increased prostaglandin production, at menstruation.

Prof. I.S. Fraser I am delighted that Professor Smith is beginning to concentrate on the regeneration of the endometrium. This is certainly an area to which relatively little attention has been paid in the past, although the morphologists have quite clearly shown regeneration taking place within the endometrium in parallel with cell destruction from as early as day 2 of menstruation, and it seems to me that this is likely to be an important mechanism in bringing menstruation to an end.

However, I suspect it is unlikely to be involved significantly in ovulatory dysfunctional bleeding, since P.J. Haynes, A.B.M. Anderson *et al.* have shown that the pattern of menstrual loss in women with ovulatory dysfunctional bleeding appears to be very much the same as normal women with up to 90% of the blood loss in the first 3 days. It would probably be more useful looking in women who had prolonged bleeding.

Mr E. Versi Coming back to the EGF story, Professor Smith showed a slide which indicated that EGF increases proliferation as does oestradiol. In another histogram he showed that the two together had a synergistic effect. If the theory about oestradiol stimulating EGF which would then have the proliferative effect was correct, then surely there would be a greater amplification. Is he not looking at two things that are happening but are dissociated?

Prof. S.K. Smith It does raise an important question as to whether EGF acts as a paracrine or as an autocrine agent. At this stage to demonstrate any effect is what is important, and we now need to go on and see whether it is an autocrine or paracrine mechanism.

Dr M.A. Lumsden   Professor Smith alluded briefly to the relationship between EGF and prostacyclin–prostaglandin production. Has he done anything with progesterone withdrawal and might this also affect EGF and therefore PG production?

Prof. S.K. Smith   We have not at this stage looked. The next step in the studies is to look at the effect of progesterone and oestradiol stimulation of EGF.

Dr D.R. Abramovich   Professor Smith showed a slide related to PKC and IP3. Has much been done on that, is it important in menstrual breakdown or is it more important in regeneration?

Prof. S.K. Smith   Clearly they are important as a part of PG production. It will obviously be important in terms of regeneration; the PI pathway is a well recognized part of the second messenger system for proliferation.

2

Prostaglandin dysfunction in dysfunctional uterine bleeding

M.C.P. Rees

INTRODUCTION

Dysfunctional uterine bleeding, or abnormal bleeding in the absence of pathology, is an important clinical problem which may lead ultimately to hysterectomy. In 1985, 18 600 hysterectomies were performed for menstrual disorders in England[1]. It is an important reason for consultation to general practitioners in that 30 per 1000 consultations are for excessive menstrual bleeding[2].

Menstrual blood loss has a skewed distribution with a mean of 35 ml and a 90th percentile of 80 ml, as found in the classic study of Hallberg *et al*, in 1966[3]. Menstrual blood loss is considered excessive if greater than 80 ml: without treatment such a loss leads to iron deficiency anaemia and constitutes objective menorrhagia. Blood losses up to 1500 ml have been measured in some women (Rees, unpublished observations).

Any examination of dysfunctional uterine bleeding must include objective blood loss measurement. It is a vital assessment since women are unreliable judges of their menstrual blood loss[4]. Only 38% of women complaining of excessive bleeding have measured losses greater than 80 ml[5]. Menstrual blood loss can be easily measured by the alkaline haematin method of Hallberg and Nilsson[6].

PROSTAGLANDINS

Abnormal prostaglandin (PG) levels have been implicated in menorrhagia since the mid-1970s when Willman and colleagues[7] reported elevated endometrial concentrations of both $PGF_{2\alpha}$ and PGE_2 during the menstrual cycle in women complaining of heavy periods. The structure, biosynthesis and role of PGs in dysfunctional uterine bleeding will be discussed. The use of prostaglandin synthase inhibitors to reduce menstrual blood loss will also be described. Recently leukotrienes, like PGs also synthesized from arachidonic acid, have been found in uterine tissues. Their role in menstrual blood loss control will also be examined.

STRUCTURE AND BIOSYNTHESIS

Prostaglandins were first isolated by Goldblatt[8] and von Euler[9] in the 1930s from accessory genital glands and human semen. The association of PGs with menstruation was first reported by Pickles *et al.*[10], who found high concentrations of $PGF_{2\alpha}$ and PGE_2 in endometrium and menstrual fluid. Later, Wiqvist and colleagues[11] demonstrated that administration of $PGF_{2\alpha}$ to women during the luteal phase resulted in menstrual bleeding.

Structure

Prostaglandins are 20-carbon polyunsaturated fatty acids containing a five membered ring with two seven and eight membered carbon side chains. They are designated prostaglandins A to I depending on the ring structure. The designations PGF_{α}, PGF_{β} differentiate alternate stereochemistries of the hydroxyl group at C9. Prostaglandins belong to the 1, 2, or 3 series depending on whether they contain one, two or three double bonds in their side chains. The principal series in mammalian tissues is the 2 series. The name thromboxane A_2 (TXA_2) was given to the unstable vasocontrictor substance formed from prostaglandin endoperoxides by platelets. This does not have the basic prostaglandin structure.

14

Biosynthesis

PG synthetic pathways have been extensively reviewed and the short description presented here is based on previous work[12]. PGs are not stored in cells but are rapidly synthesized once the substrate fatty acid precursor, arachidonic acid, becomes available to the appropriate synthetic enzymes. Arachidonic acid is not present in the free state within cells but is bound in ester linkage to phospholipids. Before PG biosynthesis can begin free arachidonic acid must be liberated from cellular phospholipids by the action of phospholipases released from lysosomes. Once released, free arachidonic acid is metabolized either through a cyclo-oxygenase-mediated pathway to PGs or by a lipoxygenase pathway to leukotrienes. Both enzyme systems have been identified in human uterine tissues[13,14].

In PG synthesis arachidonic acid is converted to the endoperoxide intermediates PGG_2 and PGH_2 through the action of the cyclo-oxygenase and peroxidase enzymes (Figure 1). Cyclo-oxygenase is present mainly in the superficial and glandular epithelium of the endometrium[15]. PGH_2 and PGG_2 are rapidly converted to the primary prostaglandins $PGF_{2\alpha}$, PGE_2 and PGD_2. PGH_2 is also converted to either TXA_2 or prostacyclin through the actions of thromboxane and prostacyclin synthetase respectively. Human uterine tissue has the capacity to produce all these substances[13,16].

The first step in leukotriene synthesis is oxygenation at C5 by the 5-lipoxygenase enzyme to form 5-hydroperoxyeicosatetraenoic acid. It is then converted to leukotriene A_4 by dehydration. This unstable allelic epoxide (LTA_4) is either hydrolysed forming leukotriene B_4 (LTB_4), or conjugated with glutathione to form leukotriene C_4 (LTC_4). In turn LTC_4 is metabolized by Y-glutamyl transpeptidase to leukotriene D_4 (LTD_4) and then by cysteinyl glycinase to LTE_4. Release of LTC_4, D_4 and E_4 has been detected in human uterine tissues[14].

PROSTAGLANDINS AND DYSFUNCTIONAL UTERINE BLEEDING

Individual PGs have differing effects on haemostasis and thus are involved in the control of menstrual blood loss volume. PGE_2, PGD_2 and prostacyclin cause vasodilatation while $PGF_{2\alpha}$ and TXA_2 cause

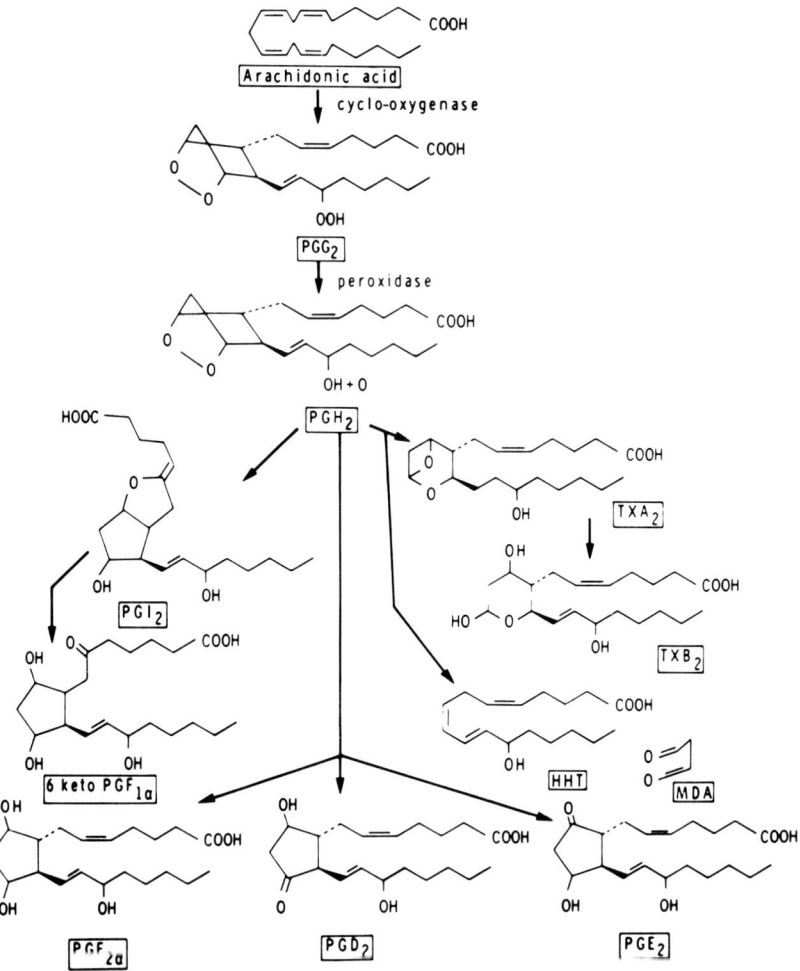

Figure 1 Prostaglandin biosynthetic pathways

vasoconstriction. Platelet aggregation is promoted by TXA_2 and inhibited by PGD_2 and prostacyclin[17,18].

Studies in relation to menstrual blood loss control have examined PGs both in menstrual fluid collected during menstruation and in endometrium and myometrium collected throughout the menstrual cycle. Most include objective measurement of menstrual blood loss.

The levels of PGs in menstrual fluid suggest increased uterine $PGF_{2\alpha}$ and PGE_2 production in menorrhagia, at least during menstruation[19]. Studies of endometrial and myometrial PGs have principally focused on

16

tissues collected at other times during the menstrual cycle using a variety of systems *in vitro* (tissue concentration, incubation, superfusion) each of which has its own limitations[20,21]. In general, PG production by uterine tissues collected throughout the menstrual cycle from menorrhagic women is not increased and does not correlate with menstrual blood loss[16]. However, in a limited number of samples obtained during the first 2 days of menstruation when the largest volume of menstrual flow occurs, the data are suggestive of a possible relationship between the volume of menstrual blood loss and $PGF_{2\alpha}$, PGE_2 and 6-keto $PGF_{1\alpha}$ release by endometrium and myometrium[16].

A shift in endometrial synthesizing capacity towards PGE_2 in menorrhagic women was originally suggested by Smith *et al.* in 1981[22] but has not been subsequently confirmed[16,23]. However, PG receptor studies suggest an altered responsiveness to the vasodilator PGE_2 in menorrhagia. In human uterine tissues, PGE_2 receptors predominate over $PGF_{2\alpha}$ receptors and are found more in the myometrium than the endometrium[25,26]. Increased concentrations of PGE receptors are present in myometrial specimens obtained from menorrhagic women and there is a direct correlation between PGE receptor concentration and menstrual blood loss[24].

Prostacyclin, the principal myometrial PG product[13,15,26], has also been examined in menorrhagia. Endometrium from women with menorrhagia is more effective than endometrium from women with normal menstrual blood loss in enhancing production of the prostacyclin metabolite 6-keto-$PGF_{1\alpha}$ in control preparations of myometrium[27]. However, increased 6-keto $PGF_{1\alpha}$ production by endometrium and myometrium *per se* in menorrhagia has not been found in other studies except during menstruation[16,28]. The suggestion that there may be increased availability of arachidonic acid in uterine tissues obtained from menorrhagic women has led to the study of phospholipase enzymes[29,30]. Phospholipase C activity was increased in endometrium from menorrhagic women but menstrual blood loss was not measured.

The leukotrienes have recently been identified in endometrium and myometrium and examined in relation to menorrhagia. However, no correlation was found between leukotriene release in either endometrium or myometrium and menstrual blood loss (Figure 2).

The implication of excessive PG levels in dysfunctional uterine bleeding has led to the use of PG synthetase inhibitors in the treatment of

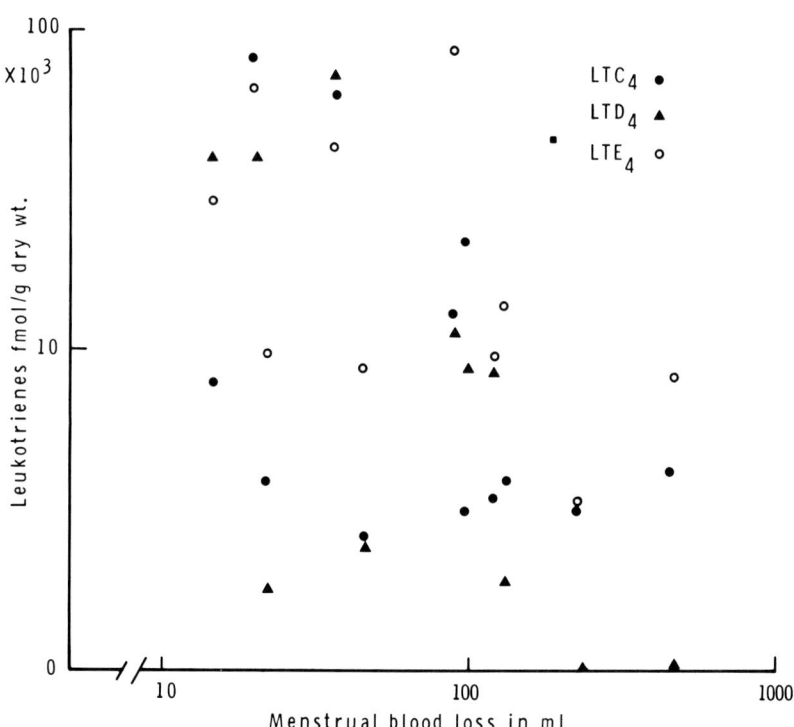

Figure 2 Leukotriene C_4 (●), leukotriene D_4 (▲) and leukotriene E_4 (O) release by endometrium in relation to menstrual blood loss

this disorder[31,32]. The effectiveness of these agents was first demonstrated by Anderson *et al.* in 1976[33]. In that study, it was observed that mefenamic acid reduced menstrual blood loss from a pretreatment mean of 119 ml to 60 ml. These findings have been confirmed in other studies[34]. Follow-up 12 to 15 months after commencing treatment showed that mefenamic acid continued to be effective in reducing menstrual blood loss[34]. Other PG synthetase inhibitors, e.g. ibuprofen, also reduce menstrual blood loss[28]. Mefenamic acid has been shown to reduce endometrial concentrations of $PGF_{2\alpha}$ and PGE_2[35]. Recently a dual mode of action has been demonstrated for fenamates. As well as reducing PG synthesis they also inhibit binding of PGE to its receptor and this additional effect, which is not shared by any other PG synthetase inhibitors, may contribute to their efficacy in the treatment of menorrhagia[36] (Figure 3).

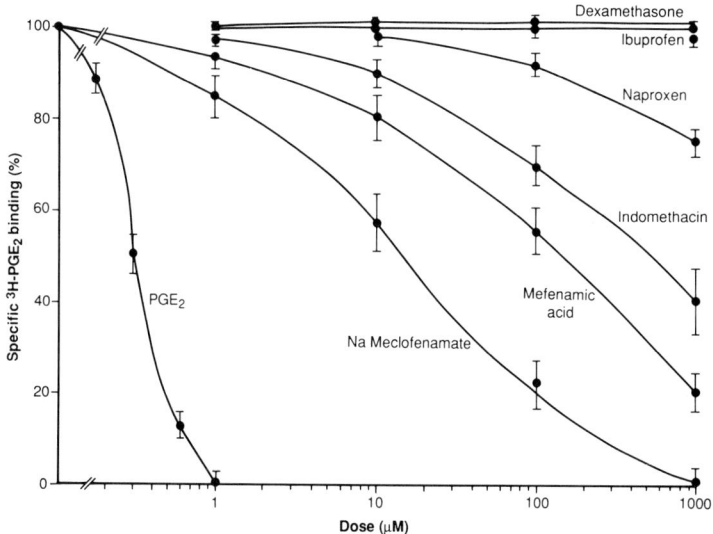

Figure 3 Inhibition of [³H]PGE₂ binding to membrane preparations of human myometrium by inhibitors of prostaglandin biosynthesis

MENSTRUAL FLUID PLATELET PROSTAGLANDIN RELEASE IN DYSFUNCTIONAL UTERINE BLEEDING

It has been apparent for many years that the mechanisms by which uterine haemostasis is achieved differ from those found in other tissue systems. Schikele in 1912 was the first to observe that menstrual fluid could be kept for several weeks without detecting any obvious clotting[37]. In most tissue systems, haemostasis consists of five somewhat overlapping phenomena: localized vasoconstriction, platelet adhesion to the lips of the wound, formation of the platelet plug, reinforcement of the platelet plug with fibrin and finally the removal of deposited material via fibrinolytic mechanisms[38].

In the uterus haemostatic plugs are only present for a limited time: few are seen beyond 20 h after the onset of menstruation and these are in any case smaller than in other tissues[39,40]. This would suggest that the contribution of haemostatic mechanisms in menstruating endometrium differs from that usually found in peripheral haemostasis.

Menstrual fluid platelets appear to be 'spent'[41]. They are unable to aggregate and metabolize arachidonic acid via the cyclo-oxygenase pathway. Furthermore, ultrastructural studies of menstrual fluid platelets have shown them to be degranulated[42]. Since degranulated platelets have also been found in endometrial haemostatic plugs it appears that menstrual fluid platelets have already been involved in uterine haemostasis before being shed[40]. The fact that B-thromboglobulin, a protein specific to human platelets which is released during thrombus formation[43], has been found in high concentrations in menstrual fluid also supports this observation[44].

Platelets obtained from the uterine vein during menstruation do not appear to be 'spent' since they aggregate normally and metabolize arachidonic acid. Therefore 'spent' platelets that would have participated in endometrial haemostasis do not seem to be returned to the systemic circulation in significant numbers[41].

A relationship between measured menstrual blood loss and platelet function has been explored. No differences were noted between venous and menstrual platelet samples obtained from women with either a light or a heavy loss[41]. Platelet abnormalities are therefore an unlikely primary factor in the aetiology of dysfunctional uterine bleeding.

CONCLUSION

It is essential that studies examining menstrual blood loss should have objective measurement of blood loss. While abnormalities of PGs have been detected in dysfunctional uterine bleeding little is known regarding their control mechanisms and future research should be directed to their examination.

ACKNOWLEDGEMENT

MCPR is a Parke Davis Lecturer.

REFERENCES

1. *Hospital Inpatient Enquiry* (1985). Table P1 (London: HMSO/OPCS)
2. *Morbidity statistics from general practice 1981–1982.* OPCS Table 13. (London: HMSO/OPCS)
3. Hallberg, L., Hogdahl, A.M., Nilsson, L. and Rybo, G. (1966). Menstrual

blood loss – a population study. *Acta Obstet. Gynecol. Scand.*, **45**, 320–51

4. Chimbira, T.H., Anderson, A.B.M. and Turnbull, A.C. (1980). Relation between measured menstrual loss and the patient's subjective assessment of loss, duration of bleeding, number of sanitary towels used, uterine weight and endometrial surface area. *Br. J. Obstet. Gynaecol.*, **87**, 603–8

5. Fraser, I.S., McCarron, G. and Markham, R. (1984). A preliminary study of factors influencing perception of menstrual blood loss volume. *Am. J. Obstet. Gynecol.*, **149**, 788–93

6. Hallberg, L. and Nilsson, L. (1964). Determination of menstrual blood loss. *Scand. J. Clin. Lab. Invest.*, **16**, 244–8

7. Willman, E.A., Collins, W.P. and Clayton, S.G. (1976). Studies in the involvement of prostaglandins in uterine symptomatology and pathology. *Br. J. Obstet. Gynaecol.*, **83**, 337–41

8. Goldblatt, M.W. (1933). A depressive substance in seminal fluid. *J. Soc. Chem. Ind. (London)*, **S2**, 1056–7

9. Von Euler, V.S. (1935). Uber die spezifische blut drucksende substanz des menslichen prostata und samenblasen secretes. *Klinische Wochenschrift*, **14**, 1182–7

10. Pickles, V.R., Hall, W.J., Best, F.A. and Smith, G.N. (1965). Prostaglandins in endometrium and menstrual fluid from normal and dysmenorrhoeic subjects. *Br. J. Obstet. Gynaecol.*, **72**, 185–95

11. Wiqvist, N., Bygdeman, M. and Kirton, K. (1971). Nonsteroidal infertility agents in the female. In Diczfalusy, E. and Barell, V.(eds), *Nobel Symposium 15 Control of human fertility*, pp. 137–67. (Stockholm: Almquist and Wiskell)

12. Green, K. (1986). Structure, biosynthesis and metabolism, In Bygdeman, M., Berger, G.S. and Keith, L.G., (eds), *Prostaglandins and their Inhibitors in Clinical Obstetrics and Gynaecology*, pp. 13–28. (Lancaster: MTP Press)

13. Demers, L.M., Rees, M.C.P. and Turnbull, A.C. (1984). Arachidonic acid metabolism by the non-pregnant human uterus. *Prost. Leuk. Med.*, **14**, 175–80

14. Rees, M.C.P., Di Marzo, V., Tippins, J.R., Morris, H.P. and Turnbull, A.C. (1987). Leukotriene release by endometrium and myometrium throughout the menstrual cycle in dysmenorrhoea and menorrhagia. *J. Endocrinol.*, **113**, 291–5

15. Rees, M.C.P., Parry, D.M., Anderson, A.B.M. and Turnbull, A.C. (1982). Immunohistochemical localisation of cyclo-oxygenase in the human uterus. *Prostaglandins*, **23**, 207–14

16. Rees, M.C.P., Anderson, A.B.M., Demers, L.M. and Turnbull, A.C. (1984). Endometrial and myometrial prostaglandin release during the menstrual cycle in relation to menstrual blood loss. *J. Clin. Endocrinol. Metab.*, **58**, 813–18

17. Lundstrom, V. (1986). The uterus. In Bygdeman, M., Berger, G.S. and Keith, L.G. (eds), *Prostaglandins and their Inhibitors in Clinical Obstetrics and Gynaecology*, pp. 59–82. (Lancaster: MTP Press)

18. Smith, B.J. (1980). The prostanoids in haemostasis and thrombosis. *Am. J. Pathol.*, **99**, 743–803

19. Wiqvist, N., Lindblom, B., Wikland, M. and Wilhelmsson, L. (1983). Prostaglandins and uterine contractility. *Acta Obstet. Gynecol. Scand., Suppl.* **113**, 23–9

20. Granstrom, E. and Samuelsson, B. (1978). Quantitative measurements of prostaglandins and thromboxanes: general considerations. In Frohlich, J.C. (ed.), *Advances in Prostaglandin and Thromboxane Research*, vol.5, pp. 1–25. (New York: Raven Press)

21. Peek, M.J., Fraser, I.S., Phillips, C.A., Resta, T.M., Blackwell, P.M. and Markham, R. (1985). The measurement of human endometrial prostaglandin production a comparison of two in vitro methods. *Prostaglandins*, **29**, 3–18

22. Smith, S.K., Abel, M.H., Kelly, R.W. and Baird, D.T. (1981). Prostaglandin synthesis in the endometrium of women with ovular dysfunctional uterine bleeding. *Br. J. Obstet. Gynaecol.*, **88**, 434–42

23. Cameron, I.T., Leask, R., Kelly, R.W. and Baird, D.T. (1987). Endometrial prostaglandins in women with abnormal menstrual bleeding. *Prost. Leuk. Med.*, **29**, 249–57

24. Adelantado, J.M., Rees, M.C.P., Lopez Bernal, A. and Turnbull, A.C. (1988). Increased uterine prostaglandin E receptors in menorrhagic women. *Br. J. Obstet. Gynaecol.*, **95**, 162–5

25. Hofman, G.E., Rao, C.V., Barrows, G.H. and Sanfilippo, J.S. (1983). Topography of human uterine prostaglandin E and F2 receptors and their profiles during pathological states. *J. Clin. Endocrinol. Metab.*, **57**, 360–6

26. Abel, M.H. and Kelly, R.W. (1979). Differential production of prostaglandins within the human uterus *Prostaglandins*, **18**, 821–8

27. Smith, S.K., Kelly, R.W., Abel, M.H. and Baird, D.T. (1981). A role for prostacyclin (PG12) in excessive menstrual bleeding. *Lancet*, **1**, 522–4

28. Makarainen, L. and Ylikorkola, O. (1986). Primary and myoma associated menorrhagia: role of prostaglandins and effect of ibuprofen. *Br. J. Obstet. Gynaecol.*, **93**, 974–8

29. Kelly, R.W., Lumsden, M.A., Abel, M.H. and Baird, D.T. (1984). The relationship between menstrual blood loss and prostaglandin production in the human: evidence for increased availability of arachidonic acid in women suffering from menorrhagia. *Prost. Leuk. Med.*, **16**, 69–75

30. Bonney, R.C. and Franks, S. (1987). Phospholipase C activity in human endometrium: its significance in endometrial pathology. *Clin. Endocrinol.*,

27, 307–20

31. Turnbull, A.C. and Rees, M.C.P. (1987). Mefenamic acid in the treatment of gynaecological disorders. *Excerpta medica*, 1–17

32. Rees, M.C.P. (1987). Menorrhagia – an algorithm. *Br. Med. J.*, **294**, 759–62

33. Anderson, A.B.M., Haynes, P.J., Guillebaud, J. and Turnbull, A.C. (1976). Reduction of menstrual blood loss by prostaglandin synthetase inhibition. *Lancet*, **1**, 774–6

34. Fraser, I.S., McCarron, G., Markham, R., Robinson, M. and Smyth, E. (1983). Long term treatment of menorrhagia with mefenamic acid. *Obstet. Gynecol.*, **61**, 109–14

35. Fraser, I.S. (1983). The treatment of menorrhagia with mefenamic acid. *Res. Clin. Forums*, 5, 93–9

36. Rees, M.C.P., Canete-Soler, R., Lopez Bernal, A. and Turnbull, A.C. (1988). Effect of fenamates on prostaglandin E receptor binding. *Lancet*, **2**, 541–2

37. Schickele, G. (1912). *Biochemische Z.*, **38**, 169–72

38. Vermylen, J. (1978). Physiology of haemostasis. In de Gaetano, G. and Garrattini, S. (eds), *Platelets: a Multidisciplinary Approach*, pp. 3–15. (New York: Raven Press)

39. Christiaens, G.C.M.L., Sixma, J.J. and Haspels, A.A. (1980). Morphology of haemostasis in menstrual endometrium. *Br. J. Obstet. Gynaecol.*, **87**, 425–32

40. Christiaens, G.C.M.L., Sixma, J.J. and Haspels, A.A. (1982). Haemostasis in menstrual endometrium; a review. *Obstet. Gynaecol. Surv.*, **37**, 281–303

41. Rees, M.C.P., Demers, L.M., Anderson, A.B.M. and Turnbull, A.C. (1984). A functional study of platelets in menstrual blood. *Br. J. Obstet. Gynaecol.*, **91**, 667–72

42. Sheppard, B.L., Dockeray, C.J. and Bonnar, J. (1983). An ultrastructural study of menstrual blood in normal menstruation and dysfunctional uterine bleeding. *Br. J. Obstet. Gynaecol.*, **90**, 259–65

43. Ludlam, C.A. and Anderton, J.L. (1978). Platelet B thromboglobulin. In Day, H.J., Harmsen, H. and Zucher, M.B. (eds). *Platelet Function Testing*, No. (NIH), 78–1087 p. 267. (Washington: US Department of Health, Education and Welfare)

44. Paton, R.C., Tindall, H., Zuzel, M. and McNicol, G.P. (1979). Haemostatic mechanisms in the normal endometrium and endometrium exposed to contraceptive steriods. In Diczfalusy, E., Fraser, I.S. and Webb, F.G.S. (eds), *Symposium on endometrial bleeding and steriodal contraception*, pp. 235–250. (Geneva: WHO)

DISCUSSION

Prof. R.W. Shaw Dr Rees has shown that mefenamates inhibit PGE binding within the tissue and PGE in my understanding is basically vasodilatory whilst PGF is a vasoconstrictor. What happens to PGF by mefenamates? Is there similar inhibition of the binding by these drugs?

Dr M.C.P. Rees The PGF receptor levels are much lower than that of PGE and binding is mainly non-specific, so we have not really looked at PGF binding.

Prof. S.K. Smith Is there no correlation between parity and menstrual blood loss? It does seen that we do not tend to see young girls complaining of menorrhagia.

Dr M.C.P. Rees We have a good population study which was done by Hallberg. He measured menstrual blood loss between the ages of 15 and 50 in a cross-sectional study. He does show that the distribution of menstrual blood loss does not change with increasing years until age 50.

3

Coagulation and electron microscopy studies in menorrhagia

B.L. Sheppard

INTRODUCTION

In recent years considerable attention has been directed towards studying the role of local uterine mechanisms in the control of normal and excessive menstrual bleeding. The control of bleeding from the uterus during menstruation is dependent on the functioning of the haemostatic system, the components of which include the blood vessels, platelets, and the coagulation and fibrinolytic enzyme systems. Biochemical and morphological examination by electron microscopy of the uterine haemostatic system has been one of the important areas of research into the mechanism of menstrual bleeding.

Menorrhagia may be associated with organic disease: the presence of an intrauterine contraceptive device (IUD) will also increase the amount and duration of menstrual bleeding[1], and electron microscopy has shown IUD-induced bleeding to be associated with a defective haemostasis in damaged blood vessels in the underlying endometrium[2-4] coupled with increased local fibrinolytic activity[5,6]. However, several studies in Europe have reported that approximately 50–60% of patients undergoing hysterectomy for menorrhagia have regular heavy menstruation with no known cause and this may be regarded as dysfunctional, or unexplained, uterine bleeding[7-9]. The observation by Haynes and colleagues[10] that in women with regular heavy periods, and no detectable pathology, ovulation usually occurs and plasma levels of oestradiol, progesterone, follicle stimulating hormone (FSH) and luteinizing hormone (LH) are similar to women with apparently normal ovulation and normal measured menstrual loss, further substantiated the need to examine local uterine mechanisms in the control of menstrual bleeding.

ENDOMETRIAL VASCULATURE

The classic observation of Markee in 1940[11] suggested that bleeding from endometrial spiral arteries accounted for 50% of total menstrual blood loss. More recent qualitative studies have shown that although arterial density is greater in the myometrium than in the endometrium there is no variation in vessel density through the normal menstrual cycle[12,13]. No significant increase is found in arterial density of the endometrium or myometrium of patients with dysfunctional uterine bleeding (Figure 1) although an increase in dilated veins is found in the functional endometrium (Figure 2). No correlation has been demonstrated between arterial density and measured menstrual blood loss[12]. In contrast, however, an increase in total blood vessel concentration has been observed in endometrium exposed to inert IUDs[14] and a decrease in

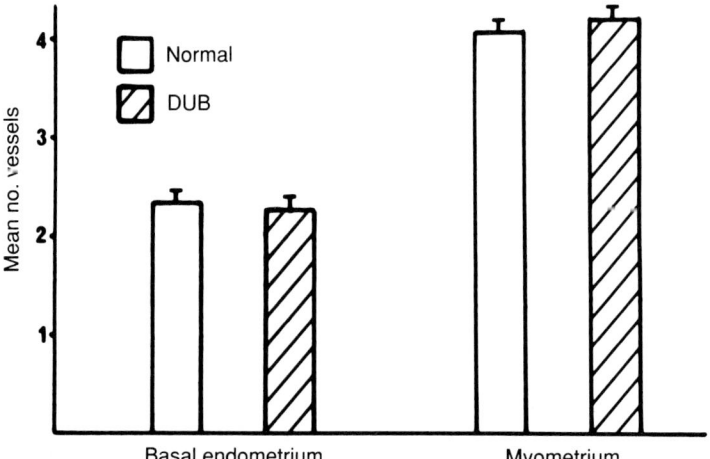

Figure 1 Number of arteries/arterioles (mean ± SEM of 12 LM fields) in the basal endometrium and adjacent myometrium in 17 control uteri (normal) and 33 uteri from patients with dysfunctional uterine bleeding (DUB). Adapted from Hourihan, Sheppard and Bonnar[13]

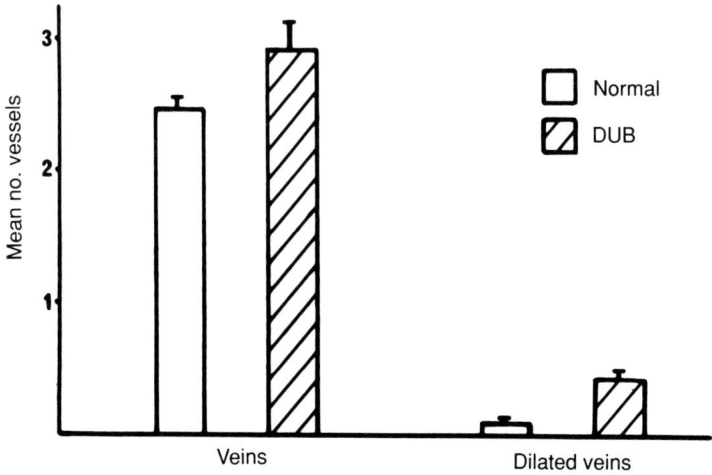

Figure 2 Number of veins and dilated veins in the functional endometrium (mean ± SEM of 12 LM fields) in 17 control uteri (normal) and 33 uteri from patients with dysfunctional uterine bleeding (DUB). A significant increase ($p < 0.05$) is found in the number of dilated veins in dysfunctional uterine bleeding. Adapted from Hourihan, Sheppard and Bonnar[13]

vessel density in endometrium exposed to the progesterone-releasing IUD[15]; whereas the former type of device is associated with an increase in menstrual bleeding, the latter is known to reduce menstrual loss[16,17].

MORPHOLOGY OF MENSTRUAL HAEMOSTASIS

Although it appears that menorrhagia in the absence of obvious pathology does not result from increased numbers of arteries, electron microscopy studies over the past decade have provided morphological evidence of a somewhat defective haemostasis in endometrial vasculature during normal menstruation[18] which is further compromised in unexplained menorrhagia[19-21]. At the onset of normal menstruation vessel lesions are seen without any haemostatic reaction (Figure 3); subsequently during the first 20 hours of menstruation, haemostatic platelet plugs are observed which are usually small (Figure 4) and seldom occlude the lumen of the endometrial blood vessels. These vessels plus thrombi are shed with the functional endometrium, and thereafter,

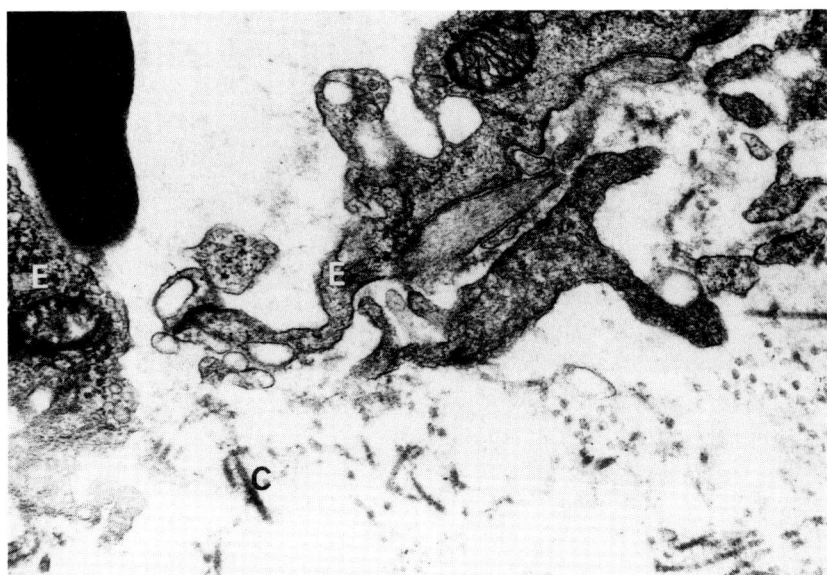

Figure 3 Part of the wall of an endometrial capillary in the premenstrual phase of the normal menstrual cycle, showing a gap between the lining endothelial cells (E) exposing the subepithelial collagen fibres (C) but without a haemostatic plug (x 36 000)

although some isolated vascular lesions may be evident, vasoconstriction is probably more important and assures haemostasis until covering of the endometrial surface by epithelium is complete.

The haemostatic events occurring in dysfunctional uterine bleeding may be considered a magnification of the mechanism of normal menstruation rather than a discrete entity. Defects in the endothelial lining of endometrial blood vessels, with and without haemostatic plugs are more common and are present for a greater number of days in patients with unexplained menorrhagia than in normal menstruation (Table 1). Whereas in normal menstruation no vascular defects may be observed after day 3 of menstruation, in dysfunctional uterine bleeding lesions are seen in endometrial blood vessels up to day 9 of the menstrual cycle[20]. The vascular defects, which ultrastructurally appear to result from contraction of endothelial cells lining the vessel walls, may be caused by histamine released, with the anticoagulant heparin, from mast cells which are found in increased numbers in the endometrium and myometrium in the late secretory phase, just prior to menstruation[21-23].

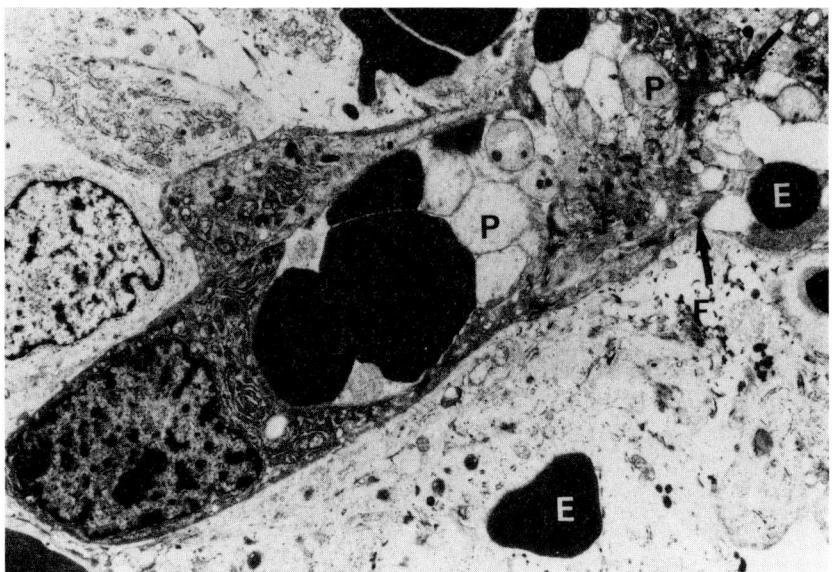

Figure 4 A capillary just below the endometrial surface in the normal menstrual cycle showing a large haemostatic plug of platelets (P) filling a gap in the endothelial lining (arrows) of the vessel wall with erythrocytes (E) and fibrin (F) in the surrounding stroma (x 6000)

Ultrastructural examination of the haemostatic plugs which form in endometrial blood vessels in unexplained menorrhagia has shown, in contrast to those seen in normal menstruation, the plugs to consist of poorly interdigitated, still granulated platelets with few fibrin fibres, and a correlation has been demonstrated between the number of these occlusive and non-occlusive haemostatic plugs and menstrual blood loss[24]. The fragility of the haemostatic plugs in unexplained menorrhagia may be partly due to diminished aggregation of the platelets or the lack of fibrin due to increased local fibrinolysis.

PLATELETS AND FIBRIN IN MENSTRUAL BLOOD

Morphological studies have shown that platelets and fibrin play a vitally important part in haemostasis in the process of menstruation. Consumption of platelet aggregates in endometrial blood vessels early in the haemostatic process of menstruation leads only to small numbers

Table 1 Morphological features in the endometrium from day 27 through menstruation to day 9 of the menstrual cycle in uteri from 12 women with normal menstruation (control) and 12 with dysfunctional uterine bleeding (DUB). Adapted from Hourihan, Sheppard and Bonner[20]

	Control			DUB	
Cycle day	*Endo. gaps*★	*Haem. plugs*†	*Cycle day*	*Endo. gaps*	*Haem. plugs*
26	–	–	26	+	–
27	+	+	29	–	–
28	–	–	30	+	–
29	–	+	32	–	+
12	+	+	1	+	+
1	+	+	2	+	+
2	+	+	2	+	–
3	–	+	3	+	+
4	–	–	4	+	+
5	–	–	7	–	+
8	–	–	9	+	+
9	–	–	9	–	+

★ Defects in the endothelial lining of endometrial blood vessels; † haemostatic plugs

being found in menstrual discharge during menstruation; the platelet count being about one-tenth of that of peripheral venous blood[25]. Although platelet thrombi may be found in 15–20% of menstrual clots (Figure 5), in our study we found 40% of clots contain no, or only isolated, single platelets[26]. The majority of menstrual platelets appear to have been exposed to an aggregating stimulus and are therefore probably spent. Ultrastructural studies of platelets collected from both the vagina and the uterus have shown they are largely devoid of granules[26,27] (Figure 6). Functional studies of platelets in menstrual fluid have found that the platelets fail to aggregate when challenged with aggregating stimuli, such as ADP and collagen, and produce no appreciable cyclo-oxygenase products from arachidonic acid[28]. In the same study no relationship was found between platelet function and menstrual blood loss, suggesting platelet abnormalities are unlikely to be a primary factor in the aetiology of dysfunctional uterine bleeding.

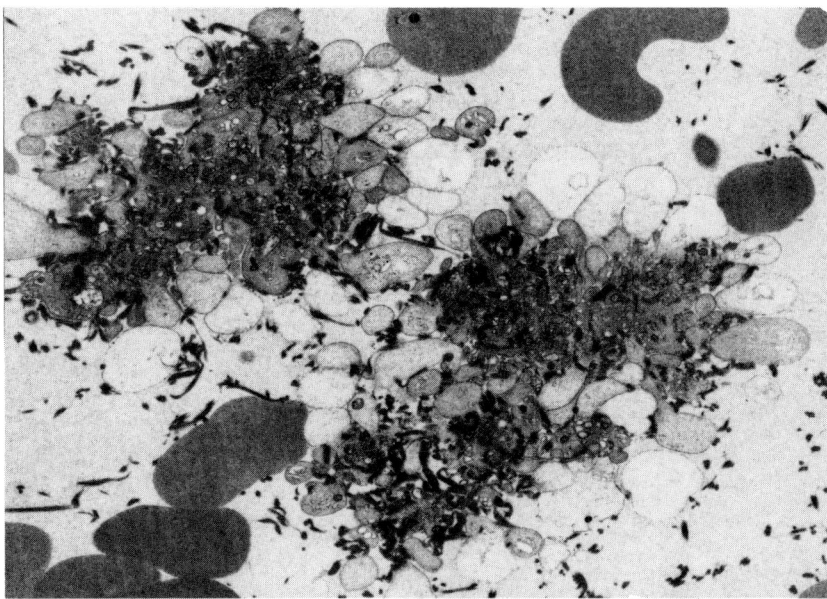

Figure 5   Electron micrograph of part of a menstrual clot containing a large platelet aggregate, electron dense fibrin fibres and erythrocytes (x 6300)

For many years it was accepted that blood clots, which are commonly found in the vagina during menstruation, were devoid of fibrin and were red cell aggregation to mucoid substances[29]. These clots become more obvious in women with excessive menstrual bleeding and our electron microscopy studies have shown that fibrin is present in 85% of menstrual clots from women both with normal menstruation and dysfunctional uterine bleeding[27]. Similar findings have also been reported in menstrual discharge before and after the insertion of an IUD[26]. These morphological studies indicate that fibrin formation occurs during the process of menstrual bleeding and that the high levels of fibrin degradation products in menstrual fluid is not solely due to a direct digestion of fibrinogen to breakdown products.

MENSTRUAL COAGULATION AND FIBRINOLYSIS

Activation of both the coagulation and fibrinolytic enzyme systems occurs during menstruation. No differences have been found in coagulation

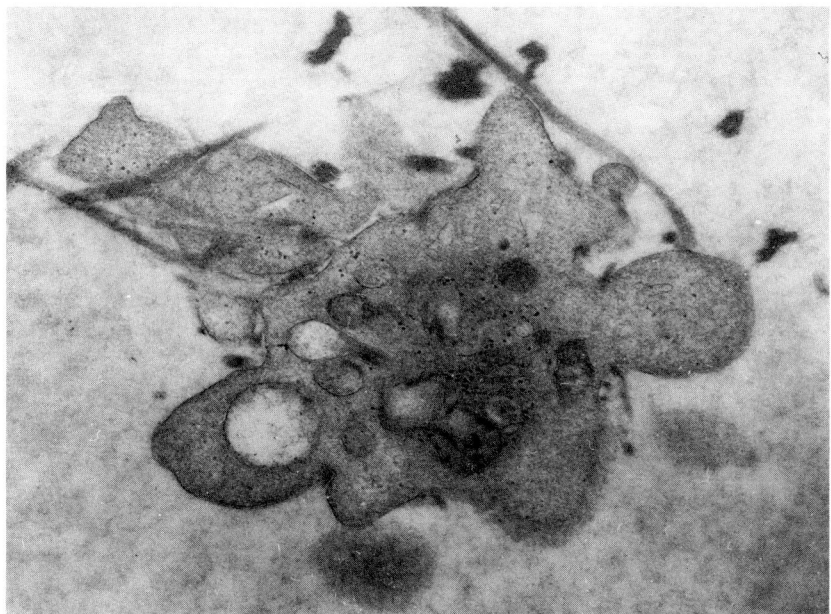

Figure 6 Electron micrograph of a single platelet in a menstrual clot. The platelet is devoid of granules, has undergone shape change in response to aggregating stimuli and appears 'spent' (x 18 000)

factors of either peripheral plasma or vaginally collected menstrual fluid between normally menstruating and menorrhagic women[30,31]. The existence of either a systemic or locally enhanced fibrinolysis in menorrhagia has been controversial[30–34]. However, evidence of the important role of increased local fibrinolytic activity in the pathogenesis of dysfunctional uterine bleeding, shown by very much higher levels of plasminogen activator in menstrual fluid of women with excessive menstrual bleeding compared to normal menstruation[35–37] (Figure 7), is further enhanced by the successful treatment with antifibrinolytic drugs[38,39], which have been shown to reduce the levels of menstrual plasminogen activator[40].

Several studies have examined coagulation and fibrinolysis of menstrual fluid, attempting to explain the mechanisms of normal and excessive menstrual bleeding. There is a general consensus of opinion that menstrual fluid contains no fibrinogen and very high levels of fibrin/fibrinogen breakdown products[41,42]. Similar levels of C_1

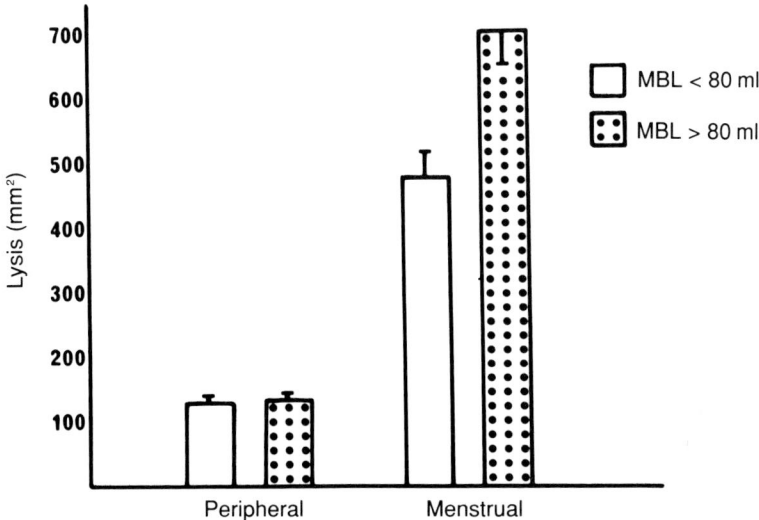

Figure 7 Comparison on fibrinolytic activity of euglobulin fractions in peripheral and menstrual blood in 20 women with normal menstrual blood loss (<80 ml MBL) and 20 women with dysfunctional uterine bleeding (>80 ml MBL). A significantly higher fibrinolytic activity is seen in the menstrual blood of women with excessive menstrual bleeding (p <0.001). Adapted from Dockeray, Sheppard, Daly and Bonnar[37]

inactivator[42], α_2 macroblobulin[31,42] and α_2 antitrypsin[42] have been found in peripheral and menstrual blood. However, compared to peripheral plasma, very low levels have been reported in menstrual fluid of activatable prothrombin[31,41], antithrombin III[36,40,42], antiplasmin[31,36,40–42], plasminogen[36,40–42], protein C[42], Factors V, VII, VIII[41] and Factor X[31]. Increased levels have been reported in menstrual fluid of Factor XII[42], free plasmin[31, 40, 41] and plasminogen activator, as measured in euglobulin fractions on a fibrin plate[31,36,40,41] of patients with excessive menstrual bleeding compared to those with normal menstruation. Recently, we have shown, using newly developed assays, a marked increase in the levels of tissue plasminogen activator antigen coupled with very low levels of plasminogen activator inhibitor in menstrual compared to peripheral plasma, which is particularly noticeable in patients with excessive menstrual bleeding[42] (Figure 8).

To date, except for the possibility of plasminogen and α_2 macroglobulin concentrations collected on the first day of menstruation[31], factors measured in menstrual or peripheral blood from

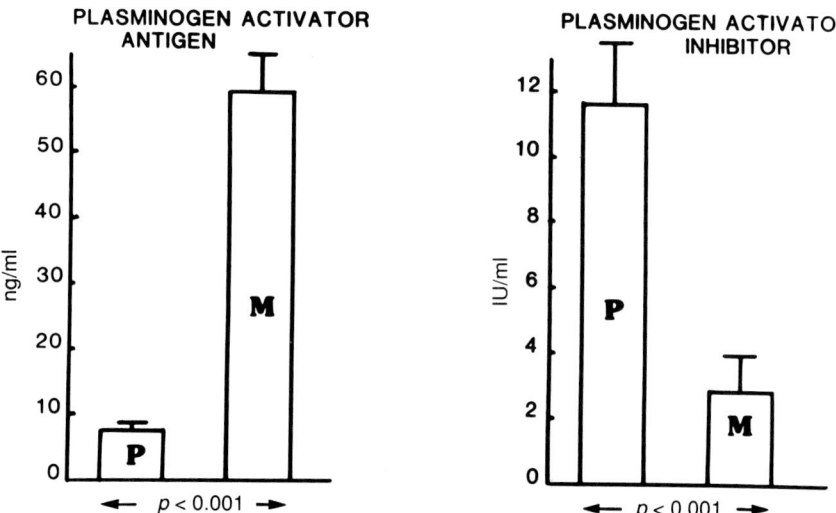

Figure 8 Tissue plasminogen activator antigen and plasminogen activator inhibitor levels in peripheral (P) and menstrual (M) blood of 12 women with known menstrual blood loss. Adapted from Daly, Sheppard, Carroll, Hennelly and Bonnar[42]

the coagulation of fibrinolytic enzyme systems have not shown any direct correlation to the degree of menstrual blood loss. Whereas in some studies the menstrual fluid was collected from the vagina[21], others collected menstrual fluid by catheter directly from the uterine cavity[35,36,40]. The glands of the cervical canal and the myometrium contain high concentrations of plasminogen activator[43–45] which may explain the conflicting reports of the relationship of plasminogen activator in menstrual fluid to the amount of menstrual blood loss[21,25,36,40]. It is also possible that menstrual fluid may not accurately reflect changes in the endometrium and myometrium of the menstruating uterus.

The finding of similar levels of plasminogen activator in peripheral plasma from women with normal menstruation to those from women with excessive menstrual bleeding suggests the higher levels of plasminogen activator found in menstrual fluid are likely to be derived from the endometrium. Indeed, earlier studies of plasminogen activator revealed high concentrations in the uterus[46,47]; extracts of secretory endometrium and endometrium from women with endometrial hyperplasia were found to contain large amounts of activator[47,48]. In women with excessive menstrual bleeding the concentration of

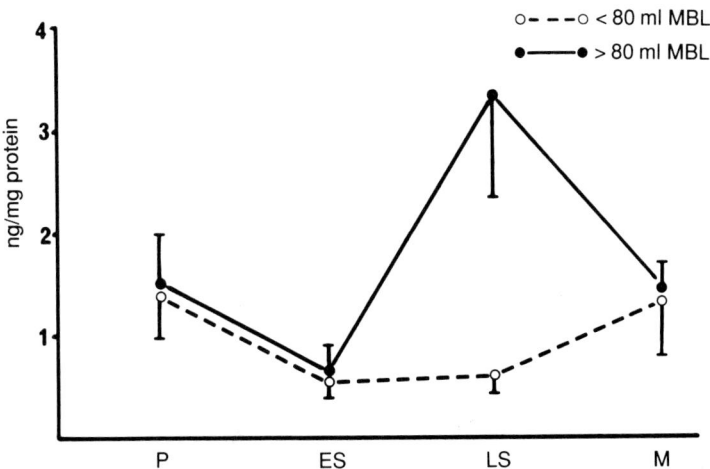

Figure 9 Tissue plasminogen activator antigen levels in extracts of endometrium from uteri removed by hysterectomy during the proliferative (P), early secretory (ES), late secretory (LS) and menstrual (M) phases of the cycle in women with normal (<80 ml MBL) and excessive (>80 ml MBL) menstrual bleeding. Adapted from Sheppard, Stack, Jordan and Bonnar[49]

plasminogen activator was found to be significantly higher when compared to women with normal menstrual loss[48]. Preliminary results in a study of endometrial and myometrial tissue extracts in our own department have shown levels of tissue plasminogen activator antigen to rise significantly more in the endometrium in the late secretory phase of the menstrual cycle in patients with excessive menstrual bleeding than in patients with normal menstrual loss[49] (Figure 9). Immunohistochemical staining of the uterine wall has shown the tissue plasminogen activator to be predominantly localized in small blood vessels of the myometrium and in spiral arteries of the endometrium in the late secretory phase of the menstrual cycle.

CONCLUSION

Both laboratory and clinical research have established that profound changes occur in the uterine haemostatic system during the process of normal menstruation which are further compromised in women with unexplained menorrhagia. Some controversy still exists as to the precise nature of these haemostatic changes, particularly in respect of their relationship to dysfunctional uterine bleeding. Divergence of findings reported in some studies may, in part, simply be due to differences in patient/study material selection or methodology. In recent years it has become increasingly evident that the objective measurement of a woman's blood loss[50] is extremely important in studies involving mechanisms of menstrual bleeding. Several studies have shown that the amount of menstrual blood loss is neither proportional to the woman's perception nor to clinical parameters, such as duration of menses, or the numbers or total weight of sanitary wear[7,51,52]. In fact as many as 60% of women attending the gynaecology out-patient clinics, complaining of excessive menstrual bleeding, may have a mean measured menstrual blood loss of less than 80 ml per cycle and be considered within the range for normal menstruation[9].

Although the precise mechanism of dysfunctional uterine bleeding still remains unclear, electron microscopy studies have shown a definite vascular defect in the endometrium, particularly in respect of haemostatic plug formation[20,21], and biochemical studies have shown a relationship between unexplained menorrhagia and increased endometrial fibrinolysis[48,49] and an increased endometrial synthesis of vasodilating and platelet aggregation inhibiting prostaglandins[53]. It is, perhaps, a little disappointing that given the striking changes in the uterine haemostatic system during menstruation, no specific factors have been isolated in menstrual fluid which relate to the degree of menstrual blood loss. However, exploration of the coagulation and fibrinolytic enzyme systems has recently been greatly facilitated by the development of new assays which may lead to the identification of more precise changes in this dynamic process. Recent studies suggest that the majority of cases of unexplained menorrhagia are due to local endometrial or myometrial dysfunction, indicating that more valuable information may be obtained by directly studying changes in components of the uterus rather than in menstrual fluid. These further studies are required to improve our understanding of the pathogenesis of dysfunctional uterine bleeding so that advances can be made in a specific treatment to restore normal menstrual function.

ACKNOWLEDGEMENTS

Some of the findings reported here are from studies supported by the Health Research Board, Ireland; the Adelaide Hospital Research Foundation, Dublin; the World Health Organisation; Kabi Vitrum, Sweden; and Warner Lambert (UK) Ltd. The collaboration of my colleagues, Prof. J. Bonnar, Dr C. J. Dockeray, Dr H. Hourihan, Dr L. Drudy, Dr M. Stack, Sister E. Carroll, Nurse B. Hennelly, Ms L. Daly and Ms M. Jordan – past and present members of the research team studying the mechanism of menstrual bleeding in the TCD Department of Obstetrics and Gynaecology, Dublin, is gratefully acknowledged.

REFERENCES

1. Guillebaud, J., Bonnar, J., Morehead, J. and Matthews, A. (1976). Menstrual blood loss with intrauterine devices. *Lancet*, **1**, 387
2. Hohman, W.R., Shaw, S.T., Macaulay, L. and Moyer, D.L. (1977). Vascular defects in human endometrium caused by intrauterine contraceptive devices. *Contraception*, **16**, 507–22
3. Sheppard, B.L. and Bonnar, J. (1980). The response of endometrial blood vessels to intrauterine contraceptive devices: an electron microscopic study. *Br. J. Obstet. Gynaecol.*, **87**, 143–54
4. Sheppard, B.L. and Bonnar, J. (1983). The effects of intrauterine contraceptive devices on the ultrastructure of the endometrium in relation to bleeding complications. *Am. J. Obstet. Gynecol.*, **146**, 829–39
5. Bonnar, J., Kasonde, J.M., Haddon, M., Hussanein, M.K. and Allington, M.J. (1976). Fibrinolytic activity in utero and bleeding complications with intrauterine devices. *Br. J. Obstet. Gynaecol.*, **83**, 160–5
6. Bonnar, J. and Sheppard, B.L. (1985). Fibrinolytic activity and intrauterine contraceptive devices. In Zatuchni, G.I., Goldsmith, A. and Sciarra, J.J. (eds). Intrauterine Contraception: Advances and Future Prospects, pp. 307–18 (Chicago: J.B. Lippincott)
7. Chimbira, T.H., Anderson, A.B.M. and Turnbull, A.C. (1980). Relation between measured menstrual loss and patient's subjective assessment of loss, duration of bleeding, number of sanitary towels used, uterine weight and endometrial surface area. *Br. J. Obstet. Gynaecol.*, **87**, 603–9
8. Rybo, G. (1982). Variations in menstrual loss. *Res. Clin. Forums*, **4**, 81–92
9. Carroll, E., Henelly, B., Sheppard, B.L. and Bonnar, J. (1989). Menstrual blood loss in patients referred to the gynaecology outpatient clinic with

excessive menstrual bleeding. *Ir. J. Med. Sci.*, **158**, 129

10. Haynes, P.J., Anderson, A.B.M. and Turnbull, A.C. (1979). Patterns of menstrual blood loss in menorrhagia. *Res. Clin. Forums*, **1**, 73–8

11. Markee, J.E. (1940). Menstruation in intraocular endometrial transplants in the rhesus monkey. *Contrib. Embryol. Carneg. Inst.*, **28**, 219–308

12. Rees, M.C.P., Dunnhill, M.S., Anderson, A.B.M. and Turnbull, A.C. (1984). Quantitative uterine histology during the menstrual cycle in relation to measured menstrual blood loss. *Br. J. Obstet. Gynaecol.*, **91**, 662–6

13. Hourihan, H.M., Sheppard, B.L. and Bonnar, J. (1986). A morphometric study of the effect of oral norethisterone and levonorgestrel in endometrial blood vessels. *Contraception*, **34**, 603–12

14. Shaw, S.T., Macaulay, L.K. and Hohman, W.R. (1979). Vessel density in endometrium of women with and without intrauterine contraceptive devices: a morphometric evaluation. *Am. J. Obstet. Gynecol.*, **135**, 202–6

15. Shaw, S.T., Macaulay, L.K., Aznar, R., Gonzalez-Angulo, A. and Roy, S. (1981). Effects of a progesterone-releasing intrauterine contraceptive device on endometrial blood vessels: a morphometric study. *Am. J. Obstet. Gynecol.*, **141**, 821–7

16. Nilsson, C.G. (1977). Comparative quantitation of menstrual blood loss with a d-Norgestral-releasing IUD and a Nova-T-copper device. *Contraception*, **15**, 379–87

17. Rybo, G. (1978). The IUD and endometrial bleeding. *J. Reprod. Med.*, **20**, 175–82

18. Christiaens, G.C.M.L., Sixma, J.J. and Haspels, A.A. (1980). Morphology of haemostasis in menstrual endometrium. *Br. J. Obstet. Gynaecol.*, **87**, 425–39

19. Sheppard, B.L. (1984). The pathology of dysfunctional uterine bleeding. *Clin. Obstet. Gynaecol.*, **11**, 227–38

20. Hourihan, H.M., Sheppard, B.L. and Bonnar, J. (1989). The morphologic characteristics of menstrual haemostasis in patients with unexplained menorrhagia. *Int. J. Gynecol. Pathol.*, **8**, 221–9

21. Sheppard, B.L., Drudy, L., Hourihan, H.M., Daly, L., Dockeray, C.J., Sharma, S.C. and Bonnar, J. (1986). Structural and functional evidence for a role of histamine in the pathogenesis of excessive menstrual bleeding. *Ir. J. Med. Sci.*, **154**, 152

22. Drudy, L., Sheppard, B.L. and Bonnar, J. (1990). Mast cells in the normal uterus and in dysfunctional uterine bleeding. (Submitted for publication)

23. Drudy, L., Sheppard, B.L. and Bonnar, J. (1990). Histamine concentration in the normal uterus and in dysfunctional uterine bleeding. (Submitted for publication)

24. Eijkeren, M.A. van, Christiaens, G.C.M.L., Geuze, J.J., Haspels, A.A. and Sixma, J.J. (1990). Morphology of menstrual haemostasis in essential menorrhagia. (In press)

25. De Merre, L.J., Moss, J.D. and Pattison, D.S. (1967). The haematologic study of menstrual discharge. *Obstet. Gynecol.*, **30**, 830–3

26. Christiaens, G.C.M.L., Sixma, J.J. and Haspels, A.A. (1981). Fibrin and platelets in menstrual discharge before and after the insertion of an intrauterine contraceptive device. *Am. J. Obstet. Gynecol.*, **140**, 793–8

27. Sheppard, B.L., Dockeray, C.J. and Bonnar, J. (1983). An ultrastructural study of menstrual blood in normal menstruation and dysfunctional uterine bleeding. *Br. J. Obstet. Gynaecol.*, **90**, 254–65

28. Rees, M.C.P., Demers, L.M., Anderson, A.B.M. and Turnbull, A.C. (1984). A functional study of platelets in menstrual fluid. *Br. J. Obstet. Gynaecol.*, **91**, 667–72

29. Beller, F.K. (1971). Observations on the clotting of menstrual blood and clot formation. *Am. J. Obstet. Gynecol.*, **111**, 535–46

30. Hahn, L., Cederblad, G., Rybo, G., Pehrsson, N.G. and Korsan-Bengtsen, K. (1976). Blood coagulation, fibrinolysis and plasma protein in women with normal and excessive menstrual blood loss. *Br. J. Obstet. Gynaecol.*, **83**, 974–80

31. Rees, M.C.P., Cederholm-Williams, S.A. and Turnbull, A.C. (1985). Coagulation factors and fibrinolytic proteins in menstrual fluid collected from normal and menorrhagic women. *Br. J. Obstet. Gynaecol.*, **92**, 1164–8

32. Cole, S.K. and Clarksson, A.R. (1972). Menstrual blood loss and fibrin degradation products. *Br. Med. J.*, **1**, 78–9

33. Rybo, G. (1966). Plasminogen activator in the endometrium. *Acta Obstet. Gynecol. Scand.*, **45**, 411–28

34. Hahn, L. and Rybo, G. (1975). Fibrinogen-fibrin degradation products in menstrual blood from women with normal and excessive menstrual blood losses. *Acta Obstet. Gynecol. Scand.*, **54**, 1–16

35. Sheppard, B.L., Dockeray, C.J., Sharma, S.C., Daly, L. and Bonnar, J. (1983). Fibrinolytic activity and prostaglandins in menstrual blood of patients with excessive menstrual bleeding. In Jespersen, J., Kluft, C. and Korsgaard, O. (eds). *Clinical Aspects of Fibrinolysis and Thrombolysis*, pp. 421–33. (Esbjerg: South Jutland University Press)

36. Bonnar, J., Sheppard, B.L. and Dockeray, C.J. (1983). The haemostatic system and dysfunctional uterine bleeding. *Clin. Res. Forums*, **5**, 27–36

37. Dockeray, C.J., Sheppard, B.L., Daly, L. and Bonnar, J. (1990). The fibrinolytic enzyme system in dysfunctional uterine bleeding following treatment with mefenamic acid and danazol. (In preparation)

38. Nilsson, L. and Rybo, G. (1967). Treatment of menorrhagia with an

antifibrinolytic agent tranexamic acid (AMCA). *Acta Obstet. Gynecol. Scand.*, **46**, 572–80

39. Bonnar, J., Guillebaud, J., Kasonde, J. and Sheppard B.L. (1980). Clinical applications of fibrinolytic inhibition in gynaecology. *J. Clin. Pathol.*, **33**, (Suppl.14), 55–9

40. Dockeray, C.J., Sheppard, B.L. and Bonnar, J. (1987). The fibrinolytic enzyme system in normal menstruation and excessive uterine bleeding and the effect of tranexamic acid. *Eur. J. Obstet. Gynecol. Reprod. Biol.*, **24**, 309–18

41. Hahn, L. (1980). Composition of menstrual blood. In Diczfalusy, E., Fraser, I.S. and Webb, F.T.C. (eds). *Endometrial Bleeding and Steroidal Contraception*, pp. 107–31 (Bath: Pitman Press)

42. Daly, L., Sheppard, B.L., Carroll, E., Hennelly, B. and Bonnar, J. (1990). Coagulation and fibrinolysis in menstrual and peripheral blood in dysfunctional uterine bleeding. *Ir. J. Med. Sci.* (In press)

43. Astrup, T. (1958). The haemostatic balance. *Thromb. Diath. Haemorrh.*, **2**, 347–57

44. Weiss, G. and Beller, F.K. (1969). Tissue activator of the fibrinolytic enzyme in the female reproductive system. *Obstet. Gynecol.*, **34**, 809–11

45. Glas-Greenwalt, P., Beller, F.K. and Astrup, T. (1971). Comparative assays of tissue plasminogen activator in myometrium, cervix and fibromyomas of the human uterus. *Am. J. Obstet. Gynecol.*, **110**, 721–5

46. Albrechtsen, O.K. (1956). The fibrinolytic activity of the human endometrium *Acta Endocrinol.*, **23**, 207–18

47. Albrechtsen, O.K. (1957). The fibrinolytic activity of the human tissue. *Br. J. Haematol.*, **3**, 284–91

48. Rybo, G. (1966). Plasminogen activators in the endometrium. II. Clinical aspects. *Acta Obstet. Gynecol. Scand.*, **45**, 429–50

49. Sheppard, B.L., Stack, M., Jordan, M. and Bonnar, J. (1990). Tissue plasminogen activator in the normal uterus and in dysfunctional uterine bleeding. *Ir. J. Med. Sci.* (In press)

50. Hallberg, L. and Nilsson, L. (1964). Determination of menstrual blood loss. *Scand. J. Clin. Lab. Invest.*, **16**, 244–8

51. Hallberg, L., Hogdahl, A., Nilsson, L. and Rybo, G. (1966). Menstrual blood loss – a population study. *Acta Obstet. Gynecol. Scand.*, **45**, 320–5

52. Fraser, I.S., McCurron, G. and Markham, R. (1984). A preliminary study of factors influencing perception of menstrual blood loss volume. *Am. J. Obstet. Gynecol.*, **149**, 788–93

53. Smith, S.K., Abel, M.H., Kelly, R.W. and Baird, D.T. (1981). Prostaglandin synthesis in the endometrium of women with ovular dysfunctional bleeding. *Br. J. Obstet. Gynaecol.*, **88**, 825–37

DISCUSSION

Dr H.P. McEwan   Do age and parity have any effect on the histology of the endometrium?

Prof. B.L. Sheppard   The short answer to that is no. The only difference that has been shown relative to parity in blood vessels of the uterus is an increase in the amount of elastic tissue in spiral arteries, with an increase with parity.

4

Phospholipases – a role in dysfunctional uterine bleeding?

R.C. Bonney, J. Higham, J.S. Beesley, H. Watson and S. Franks

INTRODUCTION

Dysfunctional uterine bleeding describes abnormal menstrual bleeding that is not explained by organic pathology. It is classified by the character of the menstrual cycle and may be ovulatory or anovulatory. Anovulatory dysfunctional uterine bleeding can occur at any age but is more frequent following menarche and during the years preceding the menopause. Anovulatory cycles result in exposure of the endometrium to stimulation by unopposed oestrogen which may give rise to abnormal endometrial development and cause dysfunctional uterine bleeding. Ovulatory dysfunctional uterine bleeding is most prevalent in parous women between the ages of 30 and 45 years and is characterized by heavy but regular menstruation. In this case, hormonal cyclicity is normal and in the absence of an explanation on the basis of endometrial abnormality, other causes must be sought.

Prostaglandins (PGs) of the 2-series synthesized by the uterus are considered to play a key role in the process of menstruation. Endometrial tissue concentrations of $PGF_{2\alpha}$, PGE_2, PG_6-keto-$F_{1\alpha}$ (the primary metabolite of PGI_2) and PGD_2 have all been shown to increase during mid-luteal and menstrual phases of the cycle[1-6]. These PGs have opposing effects on the uterus: PGE_2, PGI_2 and PGD_2 cause vasodilatation of blood vessels and anti-platelet aggregation whereas

$PGF_{2\alpha}$ causes platelet aggregation and vasoconstriction. All are therefore potential mediators in the regulation of menstrual blood loss and an imbalance in the production of one or more of these substances has been associated with dysfunctional uterine bleeding[7-9].

The rate limiting step in the synthesis of PGs of the 2-series is the liberation of free arachidonic acid from lipid precursors. Free arachidonic acid is commonly considered to originate from the hydrolysis of phospholipids by the enzyme phospholipase A_2 (PLA_2). Regulation of PLA_2 activity may therefore play a crucial role in the synthesis of PGs by the endometrium and could be implicated in dysfunctional uterine bleeding.

Two PLA_2 isoenzymes are present in human endometrium which differ with respect to pH and calcium requirements and may be regulated by different mechanisms[10]. Phospholipase A_2 type 1 appears to be of physiological importance whereas PLA_2 type 2 may have implications in endometrial pathology. For instance, PLA_2 type 2 activity is markedly higher in the endometrium of women with polycystic ovaries, a condition which is often associated with heavy and painful periods[11]. The endometrium of women with polycystic ovaries is thicker and the uterus larger than in normal subjects[12] implying a uterine abnormality with which the increase in PLA_2 type 2 activity may be associated. In the same study we were unable to show that there was any alteration in the activity of either isoenzyme in women with menorrhagia but our investigations were not supported by menstrual blood loss measurements[11].

An alternative pathway by which arachidonic acid may be generated is via the hydrolysis of phosphatidylinositol by phospholipase C (PLC) to yield inositol phosphates and diacylglycerol. Diacylglycerol may then be further hydrolysed by mono- and diacylglycerol lipases to release free arachidonic acid (Figure 1). All these enzymes are active in human endometrium and could fulfil this role[13,14].

The importance of PLA_2 and PLC in the physiology and pathophysiology of the uterus both in the normal menstrual cycle and in association with dysfunctional uterine bleeding is discussed below.

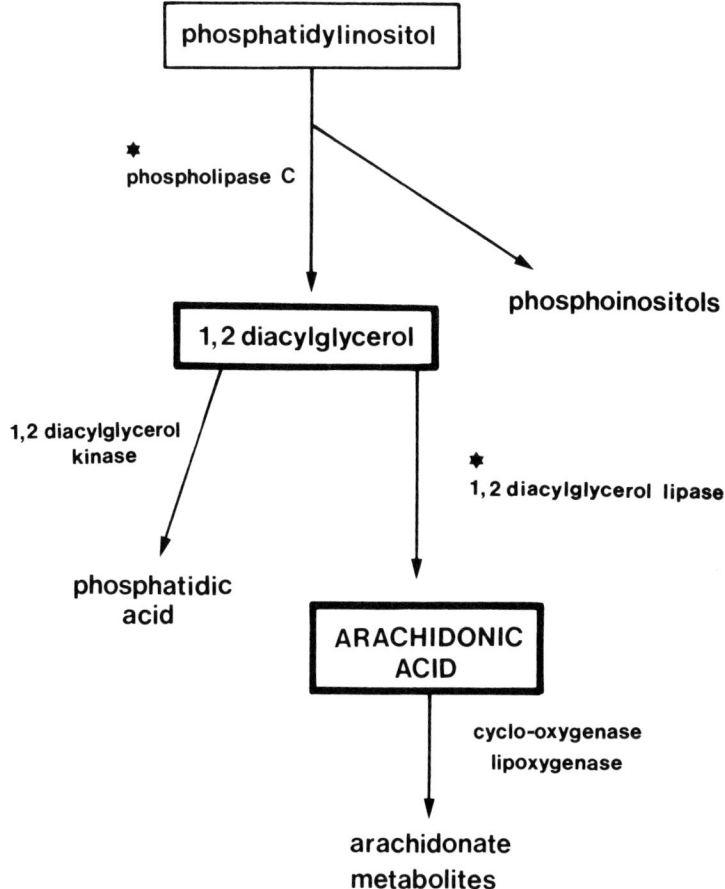

Figure 1 Pathway of arachidonic acid synthesis from phosphatidylinositol. Asterisks denote key enzymes in the pathway

PHOSPHOLIPASE A$_2$ ACTIVITY

The normal menstrual cycle

The measurement of PLA$_2$ activity in the endometrium during the menstrual cycle in women with regular ovulatory cycles has been described[10,11,15]. The original study[15] described the presence of a calcium-dependent PLA$_2$ with an optimum pH range of 7.5–9.0[15]. The activity of the enzyme was determined in homogenates of endometrium using a double isotope ratio assay which measured the release of [^{14}C]oleic acid following hydrolysis of a radiolabelled substrate, 1-palmitoyl-2[1-^{14}C] oleoyl phosphatidylcholine. Phospholipase A$_2$ activity increased during the proliferative phase to reach a maximum in the early secretory phase, 2–4 days following ovulation, thereafter declining as the secretory phase progressed to return to low levels of activity at menstruation. The profile was concomitant with an oestrogenic stimulation of PLA$_2$ activity during the proliferative phase followed by an inhibitory effect of progesterone with the progression of the luteal phase. A similar relationship between ovarian steroids and PLA$_2$ activity was demonstrated by Downing and Poyser[16] in guinea-pig endometrium during the oestrous cycle.

The decline in PLA$_2$ activity in the endometrium at the time of menstruation did not correlate with the increase in concentrations of PGs reported in the literature[1] and suggested that there may be other phospholipases present, possibly of lysosomal origin, which might be a more important trigger for menstruation. Since lysosomal phospholipases are frequently calcium independent and more active at an acidic pH, further studies were carried out. Removal of calcium from the assay medium altered the pH profile of PLA$_2$ activity and revealed a peak of activity at pH 7 which was absent when 5 mM calcium was added. By using preparations of isolated glands and stromal cells it was possible to demonstrate the presence of two distinct PLA$_2$ isoenzymes in the endometrium. Two isoenzymes of PLA$_2$ have now been described: a calcium-dependent enzyme with an optimum pH range of 7.5–9.0 which is located in the glandular component of the endometrium (PLA$_2$ type 1) and a calcium-independent enzyme with an optimum pH of 7.0 which is present in stromal cells (PLA$_2$ type 2)[10]. Phospholipase A$_2$ type 2 activity has subsequently been demonstrated in myometrium[17].

Measurement of both PLA$_2$ isoenzymes in endometrium throughout the menstrual cycle in women with normal ovulatory cycles demonstrated that whereas PLA$_2$ type 1 activity is subject to ovarian cyclicity[10,15], PLA$_2$ type 2 activity is not. The range in PLA$_2$ type 2 activity was wide and there was no apparent correlation with the stage of the menstrual cycle[10]. Again a direct association between PLA$_2$ type 2 activity and the profiles of tissue concentrations of PGs reported by others[1] was not evident.

46

Dysfunctional uterine bleeding

Do women with ovulatory dysfunctional uterine bleeding have a different profile of either PLA_2 type 1 or type 2 activity compared with those with normal menstrual blood loss? In an earlier study we attempted to answer the question and concluded that they did not[11]. The limitation of the study was however, that menstrual blood loss measurements were not available. Since there is considerable evidence to demonstrate that women do not make accurate subjective assessments of their own menstrual blood loss[16] it was necessary to confirm our findings in a further study which included an objective assessment of menstrual blood loss. The results of the study are reported below.

Endometrial tissue was obtained by vabra curettage or D & C from women with regular ovulatory cycles who presented with the complaint of heavy and regular menstrual bleeding. Menstrual blood loss was measured by the method of Hallberg and Nilsson[19] in two cycles and was classified as menorrhagia if in excess of 80 ml per period. The women included in the study had no other pathology, were ovulating regularly, had normal ovaries (as evidenced by ultrasonography), normal endocrine profiles and were not taking any medication at the time of the study. A control group was recruited from patients complaining of menorrhagia who were found to have normal blood loss and from those presenting for laparoscopic clip sterilization or being investigated for unexplained infertility later ascribed solely to tubal defects. They had no other pathology. Menstrual blood loss was always less than 40 ml per month, cycles were regular and the ovaries normal. Endometrium was dated by histology and assigned to the appropriate stage of the menstrual cycle. Phospholipse A_2 activity (types 1 and 2) was assayed as described[11,15] except that the substrate used was 1-stearoyl-2-[1-^{14}C]arachidonyl phosphatidylcholine which was considered to be physiologically more appropriate that the 2-oleoyl derivative. A prior comparison of PLA_2 activity measured in endometrial homogenates using the two substrates revealed that PLA_2 type 1 had a preference for the 2-archidonyl substrate (a doubling in the rate of hydrolysis) whereas PLA_2 type 2 did not.

There was a significant increase in PLA_2 type 1 activity during the secretory phase of the menstrual cycle in both women with normal blood loss and in those with menorrhagia ($p < 0.001$) and no difference between the two groups of subjects. The results are shown in Figure 2.

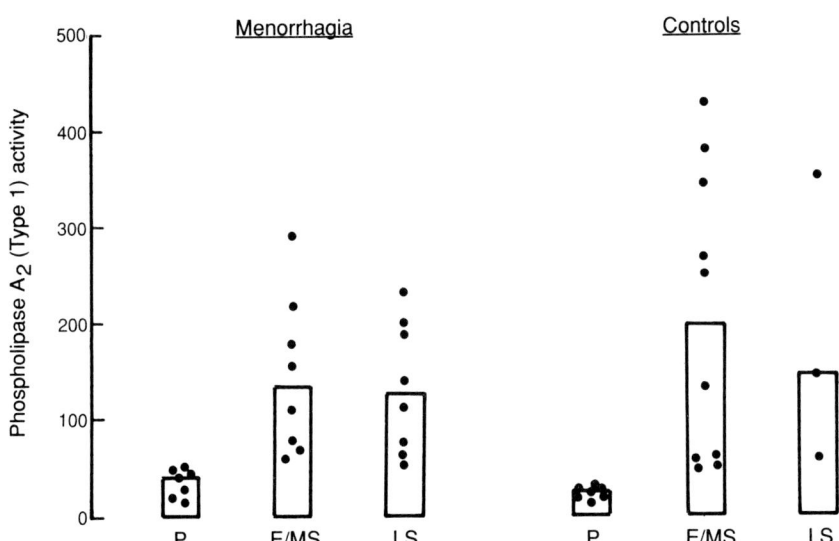

Figure 2 Phospholipase A_2 type 1 activity in endometrium with respect to the stage of the menstrual cycle in women with menorrhagia and in women with normal menstrual blood loss (controls). The data are presented as individual observations (each an average of duplicate estimations) and the median of each group is presented as a vertical bar. Phospholipase A_2 activity is expressed as pmol arachidonic acid released per mg protein per min. Abbreviations: P, proliferative phase; E/MS, early and mid-secretory phase; LS, late secretory phase. Statistical analysis: (Mann–Whitney 'U' test) menorrhagia subjects: P vs E/MS, $p < 0.001$; P vs LS, $p < 0.001$; control group: P vs E/MS, $p < 0.001$

Phospholipase A_2 type 2 activity was also significantly higher in the early/mid-secretory phases of the cycle compared with that of the proliferative phase both in women with normal blood loss ($p < 0.02$) and in those with ovulatory menorrhagia ($p < 0.01$). Again there was no difference between the two groups (Figure 3). In women with ovulatory menorrhagia there was also an increase in PLA_2 type 2 activity in late secretory phase tissue ($p < 0.05$) compared with the proliferative phase but there were too few data for a similar comparison in the control group. The study demonstrates that with respect to the activity of both PLA_2 type 1 and PLA_2 type 2 there is no difference between women with normal menses and those with ovulatory dysfunctional uterine bleeding. These observations lend weight to our earlier study, referred to above, conducted in the absence of menstrual blood loss measurements where there was also no difference between the two groups[11].

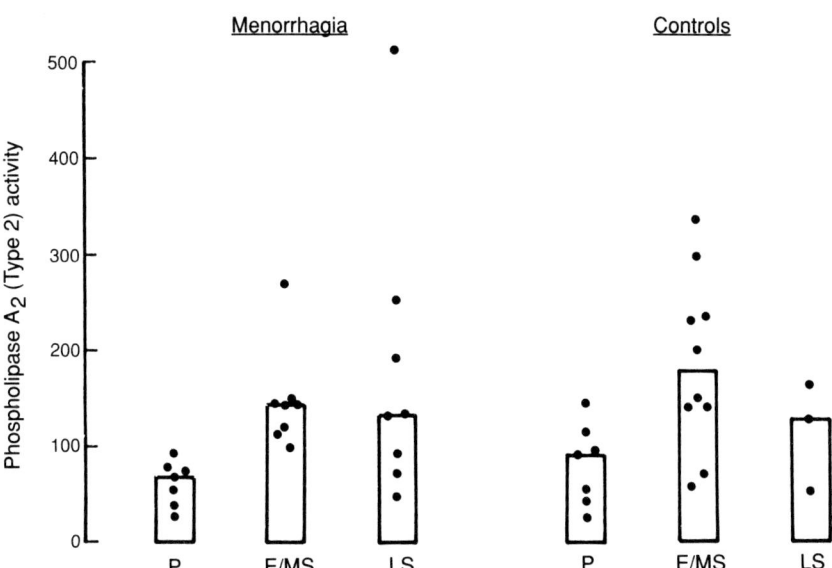

Figure 3 Phospholipase A_2 type 2 activity in endometrium with respect to the stage of the menstrual cycle in women with menorrhagia compared with women with normal menstrual blood loss (controls). The data are presented as individual observations (each an average of duplicate estimations) and the median of each group is presented as a vertical bar. Phospholipase A_2 activity is expressed as pmol arachidonic acid released per mg protein per min. Abbreviations: P, proliferative phase; E/MS, early and mid-secretory phase; LS, late secretory phase. Statistical analysis: (Mann–Whitney 'U' test) menorrhagia subjects: P vs E/MS, $p < 0.001$; P vs LS, $p < 0.05$; control group: P vs E/MS, $p < 0.02$

Fibroids and menorrhagia

Fibroids constitute a common uterine disorder which is frequently associated with menorrhagia although these benign tumours could be incidental to and not the cause of bleeding. The aetiology of fibroids is not well understood but it is recognized that their development is influenced by changes in ovarian function and that unopposed oestrogen has a growth promoting effect[20,21]. Fibroids synthesize PGI_2[22] which could contribute to an imbalance in PG production and be responsible in part for the menorrhagia and dysmenorrhoea associated with this condition.

Phospholipase A_2 activity was measured in proliferative phase endometrium in a limited number of women who presented with

Table 1 The activity of phospholipase A$_2$ in proliferative phase endometrium in women with menorrhagia ($n=7$)

	PLA$_2$ type 1		PLA$_2$ type 2★	
	Median	Range	Median	Range
Control group	24.1	14.4–30.5	90.0	24.9–146.4
Fibroids/menorrhagia	34.1	18.2–51.4	147.8	39.7–405.9
Ovulatory menorrhagia	40.4	18.8–50.0	68.8	30.7– 93.8

★ pmol/mg protein/min; no significant differences (Mann–Whitney 'U' test)

menorrhagia and were subsequently found to have fibroids. The results are presented in Table 1. There was no significant difference between the control group and the group with fibroids with respect to the activity of either PLA$_2$ type 1 or PLA$_2$ type 2. There was also no difference between women with ovulatory menorrhagia and those with fibroids and menorrhagia. However, the numbers in the study were too few and the variation between individual subjects was too great for a satisfactory conclusion to be drawn from the data.

The myometrium has a limited ability to synthesize PGs compared with the endometrium and has been shown to produce predominantly PGI$_2$[23] which has potent antiaggregatory and vasodilatory effects. However, if the myometrial mass is taken into account then the amount of PGI$_2$ produced could be important in the regulation of uterine bleeding. The myometrium possesses a single PLA$_2$ enzyme which appears to be identical to PLA$_2$ type 2 activity of the endometrium. The enzyme has been measured in the myometrium of 41 women presenting with menorrhagia, 22 of whom also had fibroids[17] and it was shown that there was no difference in activity between the two phases of the cycle. However, myometrial PLA$_2$ activity was significantly higher when the uterus contained fibroids ($p<0.01$) (Table 2). There was also an age associated increase in PLA$_2$ type 2 activity in the myometrium of women in the 41–50 age group which was not related to the presence of fibroids (Table 3). The increase in activity is most likely to be due to an increase in the incidence of anovulatory cycles and the action of unopposed oestrogen on the myometrium in the women in this age group.

Table 2 The association between myometrial PLA_2 activity (nmol product/mg protein/h) and fibroids

	n	Median	Range
Fibroids	22	11.3★	2.2–30.9
No fibroids	19	6.9★	0.3–25.8

Significantly different ★$p<0.01$, Mann–Whitney 'U' test

Table 3 The association between myometrial PLA_2 activity (nmol product/mg protein/h), age of subject and fibroids in women with menorrhagia

Age (yr)	All subjects			Subjects without fibroids		
	Median	Range	n	Median	Range	n
33–40	4.7★★	0.3– 6.9	13	4.7★	0.3– 7.6	9
41–50	11.3★★	2.2–30.9	21	7.8★	2.2–25.8	11
51–55	8.7	2.5–17.7	7	6.9	3.9–11.5	4

Significantly different: ★$p<0.01$, ★★$p<0.001$; Mann–Whitney 'U' test

Polycystic ovaries

In a preliminary study it was observed that there was a marked increase in PLA_2 type 2 activity in the endometrium of women with polycystic ovaries although PLA_2 type 1 activity was no different from that seen in women with normal ovaries[11]. Polycystic ovaries are associated with an enlarged uterus and a thickened endometrium which suggests a uterine abnormality with which the increase in PLA_2 activity could be associated. Since women with polycystic ovaries may also present with menstrual difficulties, including menorrhagia, we report here on the activity of PLA_2 types 1 and 2 in the endometrium of women with polycystic ovaries compared with that of a control group. The study was restricted to women with ovulatory polycystic ovaries in order to exclude those with endometrial abnormalities due to anovulation. The subjects were identified by ultrasonagraphy of the ovaries; confirmation of ovulation was obtained by serial ultrasound scans and timed serum progesterone

51

determinations. Endometrium was obtained by endometrial biopsy or D & C and PLA_2 activity measured as indicated above. The data obtained are compared with those of the control group (as described above for the menorrhagia study) and presented in Figures 4 and 5. In women with polycystic ovaries as in the control group, PLA_2 type 1 activity was significantly higher in secretory phase tissue than in proliferative phase tissue ($p < 0.001$). There was no significant difference between the two groups of women (Figure 4). As shown in Figure 5, the activity of PLA_2 type 2 in the control group was also significantly higher in the secretory phase compared with that of the proliferative phase ($p < 0.01$). However, in women with polycystic ovaries, the activity of PLA_2 type 2 was increased in the proliferative phase to the level of that of the secretory phase and no difference was observed between the two phases of the cycle. Accordingly, PLA_2 type 2 activity was significantly higher in the proliferative phase of women with polycystic ovaries compared with that of the control group ($p < 0.001$). There was no difference between the

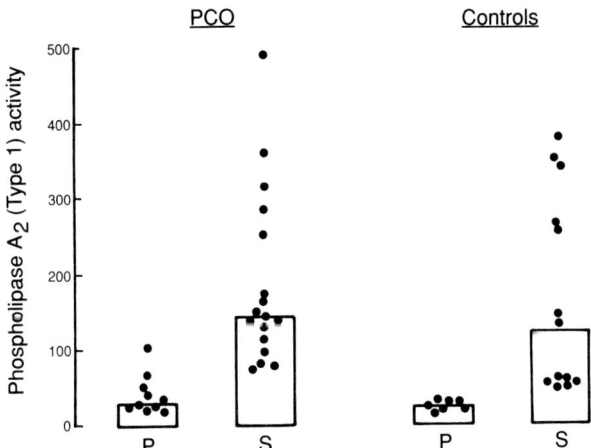

Figure 4 Phospholipase A_2 type 1 activity in endometrium with respect to the stage of the menstrual cycle in women with ovulatory polycystic ovaries (PCO) compared with women with normal ovaries (controls). The data are presented as individual observations (each an average of duplicate estimations) and the median of each group is presented as a vertical bar. Phospholipase A_2 activity is expressed as pmol arachidonic acid released per mg protein per min. Abbreviations: P, proliferative phase; S, secretory phase. Statistical analysis; (Mann–Whitney 'U' test) PCO subjects: P vs S, $p < 0.001$; control group: P vs S, $p < 0.001$

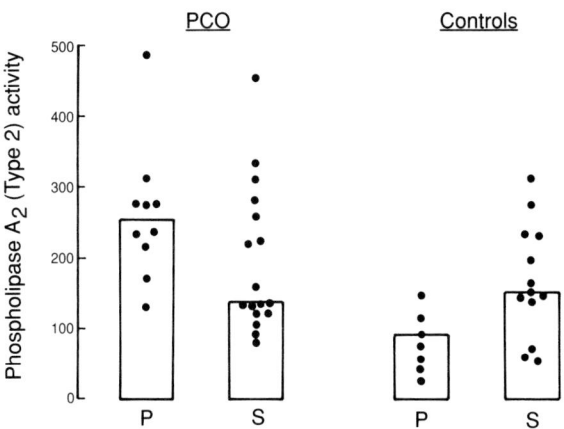

Figure 5   Phospholipase A_2 type 2 activity in endometrium with respect to the stage of the menstrual cycle in women with ovulatory polycystic ovaries (PCO) compared with women with normal ovaries. The data are presented as individual observations (each an average of duplicate estimations) and the median of each group is presented as a vertical bar. Phospholipase A_2 activity is expressed as pmol arachidonic acid released per mg protein per min. Abbreviations: P, proliferative phase; S, secretory phase. Statistical analysis: (Mann–Whitney 'U' test) PCO subjects: P vs S, no significant difference; control group: P vs S, $p < 0.05$; PCO subjects vs control subjects: proliferative phase, $p < 0.001$, secretory phase, no significant difference

secretory phases of the two groups. These data contrast with those described above for women with ovulatory menorrhagia and suggest that increased PLA_2 type 2 activity seen in the endometrium of women with polycystic ovaries may be related to the uterine abnormality which is associated with this condition. There is a predisposition to early recurrent miscarriage in women with ovulatory polycystic ovaries which suggest that the abnormality may have important clinical implications[24].

PHOSPHOLIPASE C ACTIVITY AND DYSFUNCTIONAL UTERINE BLEEDING

The activity of PLC may be monitored by measuring the accumulation of water soluble products (myoinositol phosphate) arising from the hydrolysis of 1-3-phosphatidyl-[2-³H]inositol[14].

In a previous study[14], the activity of PLC in endometrium was shown to be independent of the stage of the menstrual cycle both in women with normal menses and in those complaining of menorrhagia. It was also shown that, in women complaining of menorrhagia, there was a significant increase in PLC activity in both the proliferative and secretory phases of the cycle. The study was, however, limited by the absence of menstrual blood loss measurements. Confirmation of these results with the added support of menstrual blood loss measurements is now presented in Table 4. Two other groups are included in the present study, namely, women with menorrhagia associated with fibroids, and women with polycystic ovaries. It is of interest to note that the group with ovulatory menorrhagia had significantly higher levels of PLC activity than all other groups ($p < 0.05$). These findings are of interest in that they confirm previous reported data and that the increased activity is confined to the group with ovulatory menorrhagia. It should be borne in mind, however, that the activity of PLC only represents the first step in the pathway and that the generation of arachidonic acid will also depend on the activity of other key enzymes, notably mono- and diacylglycerol lipase. Nevertheless, the difference observed in women with ovulatory menorrhagia presents an interesting observation.

CONCLUSION

These studies emphasise the relevance of phospholipases in the physiology and pathophysiology of the uterus. Phospholipase A_2 type 1 activity appears to be confined to the endometrial glands and is not increased in uterine disorders or where there is an ovarian abnormality,

Table 4 Phospholipase C activity (nmol inositol phosphate released/mg protein/min) in endometrium

	Median	*Range*	*n*
Control group	6.1	0.4–13.5	17
Ovulatory menorrhagia★	8.2	3.2–21.7	17
Polycystic ovaries	4.8	1.6–14.7	10
Fibroid-associated menorrhagia	6.1	3.5–13.7	10

★ Significantly higher, $p < 0.05$ versus other groups (Mann–Whitney 'U' test)

e.g. in women with polycystic ovaries. It is low at menstruation which might be expected in a tissue which has become necrotic and may be more important in the establishment of implantation rather than in the mechanism of menstruation. Phospholipase A_2 type 2 activity on the other hand, appears to have some relevance to uterine pathology especially in association with polycystic ovaries. The underlying cause of the uterine abnormality found in women with ovulatory polycystic ovaries is not known but the likelihood is that there is an endocrine defect which involves steroids, i.e. oestrogens or androgens. Growth factors such as epidermal growth factor (EGF) or transforming growth factor α (TGFα) may also play a part, since oestrogens have been shown to increase EGF receptors in the uterus[25,26] and uterine growth is mediated by EGF[27]. Epidermal growth factor also stimulates arachidonic acid release from prelabelled endometrial glands[28] thus offering an important link between abnormal uterine growth and PLA_2 activity. The relevance of PLA_2 type 2 activity to dysfunctional uterine bleeding is difficult to assess. There is no apparent increase in activity in the endometrium of women with menorrhagia but this does not preclude the possibility that there is an increase in the availability of arachidonic acid as a result of increased enzyme activation as opposed to enzyme synthesis. The myometrium should also be taken into account since the major PG synthesized by this tissue is PGI_2 which has potent vasodilatory and anti-aggregatory properties. Furthermore, the capacity of the tissue to generate arachidonic acid and to synthesize PGs far exceeds that of the endometrium. It is possible therefore that an abnormality of the myometrium rather than the endometrium could cause an increase in PLA_2 activity and be in turn the cause of dysfunctional uterine bleeding.

The increase in PLC activity in women with ovulatory menorrhagia is of interest and offers a direction for further research, since without knowledge of subsequent events in the pathway one cannot predict the importance of these findings.

ACKNOWLEDGEMENTS

The work is supported by St. Mary's Hospital Save the Baby Fund, Birthright and the Wellcome Trust.

REFERENCES

1. Downie, J., Poyser, N.L. and Wunderlich, M. (1974). Levels of prostaglandins in human endometrium during the normal menstrual cycle. *J. Physiol.*, **236**, 465–72

2. Maathuis, J. B. and Kelly, R.W. (1978). Concentrations of prostaglandins $F_{2\alpha}$ and E_2 in the endometrium throughout the human menstrual cycle, after the administration of clomiphene or an oestrogen-progestogen pill and in early pregnancy. *J. Endocrinol.*, **77**, 361–71

3. Willman, E.A., Collins, W.P. and Clayton, S.G. (1976). Studies in the involvement of prostaglandins in uterine symptomatology and pathology. *Br. J. Obstet. Gynaecol.*, **83**, 337–41

4. Singh, E.J., Baccarini, I.M. and Zuspan, F.P. (1975). Levels of prostaglandins $F_{2\alpha}$ and E_2 in human endometrium during the menstrual cycle. *Am. J. Obstet. Gynecol.*, **121**, 1003–6

5. Rees, M.C.P., Anderson, A.B.M., Demers, L.M. and Turnbull, A.C. (1984). Endometrial and myometrial prostaglandin release during the menstrual cycle in relation to menstrual blood loss. *J. Clin. Endocr. Metab.*, **58**, 813–18

6. Rees, M.C.P. and Kelly, R.W. (1986) Prostaglandin D_2 release by endometrium and myometrium. *Br. J. Obstet. Gynaecol.*, **93**, 1078–82

7. Smith, S.K., Abel, M.H., Kelly, R.W. and Baird, D.T. (1981). Prostaglandin synthesis in the endometrium of women with ovular dysfunctional uterine bleeding. *Br. J. Obstet. Gynaecol.*, **88**, 434–42

8. Smith, S.K., Abel, M.H., Kelly, R.W. and Baird, D.T. (1981). A role for prostacyclin (PGI_2) in excessive menstrual bleeding. *Lancet*, **1**, 522–4

9. Smith, S.K., Abel, M.H., Kelly, R.W. and Baird, D.T. (1982). The synthesis of prostaglandins from persistent proliferative endometrium. *J. Clin. Endocr. Metab.*, **55**, 284–9

10. Bonney, R.C., Qizilbash, S.T. and Franks, S. (1987). Endometrial phospholipase A_2 enzymes and their regulation by steroid hormones. *J. Steroid Biochem.*, **27**, 1057–64

11. Bonney, R.C. and Franks, S. (1988). The activity of calcium dependent and calcium independent phospholipase A_2 in normal endometrium and in endometrium of women suffering from menorrhagia and polycystic ovary syndrome. *Gynecol. Endocrinol.*, **2**, 131–8

12. Adams, J., Franks, S., Polson, D.W., Mason, H.D., Abdulwahid, N., Tucker, M., Morris, D.V., Price, J. and Jacobs, H.S. (1985). Multifollicular ovaries: clinical and endocrine features and response to pulsatile gonadotropin releasing hormone. *Lancet*, **2**, 1375–80

13. Bonney, R.C. and Franks, S. (1988). Hydrolysis of phosphatidylinositol by

human endometrium: modulating effects of steroids on arachidonic acid and 1,2-diacylglycerol release. *J. Endocrinol.*, **117**, 309–14

14. Bonney, R.C. and Franks, S. (1987). Phospholipase C activity in human endometrium: its significance in endometrial pathology. *Clin. Endocrinol.*, **27**, 307–20

15. Bonney, R.C. (1985). Measurement of phospholipase A_2 activity in human endometrium during the menstrual cycle. *J. Endocrinol.*, **107**, 183–9

16. Downing, I. and Poyser, N.L. (1983). Estimation of phospholipase A_2 activity in guinea-pig endometrium on days 7 and 15 of the oestrous cycle. *Prost. Leuk. Med.*, **12**, 107–17

17. Bonney, R.C. and Wong, W. (1988). The measurement of phospholipase A_2 activity in human myometrium: physiological and pathological implications. *Prost. Leuk., Essential Fatty Acids*, **34**, 1–8

18. Fraser, I.S., McCarron, G. and Markham, R. (1984). A preliminary study of factors influencing perception of menstrual blood loss volume. *Am. J. Obstet. Gynecol.*, **149**, 788–93

19. Hallberg, L. and Nilsson, I. (1964). Determination of menstrual blood loss. *Scand. J. Clin. Lab. Invest.*, **16**, 244–8

20. Miller, N.F. and Ludovici, P.P. (1955). On the origin and development of uterine fibroids. *Am. J. Obstet. Gynecol.*, **70**, 720–40

21. Goldzieher, J.W., Maqueo, M., Ricaud, L., Aguilar, J.A. and Canales, E. (1966). Induction of degenerative changes in uterine myomas by high-dosage progestin therapy. *Am. J. Obstet. Gynecol.*, **96**, 1078–87

22. Rees, M.C.P. and Turnbull, A.C. (1985). Leiomyomas release prostaglandins. *Prost. Leuk. Med.*, **18**, 65–8

23. Yamaguchi, M. and Mori, N. (1987). Prostaglandin production by human myometrium uterine cervix and leiomyoma. *Prost. Leuk. Med.*, **29**, 107–12

24. Sagle, M., Bishop, K., Ridley, N., Alexander, F.M., Michel, M., Bonney, R.C., Beard, R.W. and Franks, S. (1988). Recurrent early miscarriage and polycystic ovaries. *Br. Med. J.*, **297**, 1027–8

25. Mukku, V.R. and Stancel, G.M. (1985). Regulation of epidermal growth factor receptor by oestrogen. *J. Biol. Chem.*, **260**, 9820–3

26. Taketani, Y. and Mizuno, M. (1988). Cyclic changes in epidermal growth factor receptor in human endometrium during menstrual cycle. *Endocrinol. Jpn.*, **35**, 19–25

27. Tomooka, Y., DiAugustine, R.P. and McLachlan, J.A. (1986). Proliferation of mouse uterine epithelial cells *in vitro*. *Endocrinology*, **118**, 1011–18

28. Beesley, J.S., Franks, S. and Bonney, R.C. (1989). The effect of calcium ionophore (A23187) and epidermal growth factor on the release of arachidonic acid from human endometrial cells in culture. *J. Endocrinol.*, **123** Suppl., 121

DISCUSSION

Prof. S.K. Smith I am very interested in the growth factor effects that were described. Is this simply release of arachidonic acid, or is it possible to say at this stage whether it seems to be a PLA_2 or PLC effect of EGF?

Dr R.C. Bonney I am wondering about that. These are very new studies obviously. With this study we used ionophore as well and the result we obtained was in the presence of ionophore. When we came to analyse the phospholipids we found that with ionophore alone there was a release from phosphatidylcholine, and if we added the EGF the additional release we got from the phospholipids was from phosphatidyl inositol. So it looked almost as though the ionophore was setting something up which was then enabling the EGF to work, but the release was coming from two separate pools.

Dr D.R. Abramovich Is there any physiological difference between $PLA_2(1)$ and $PLA_2(2)$?

Dr R.C. Bonney That I do not know at the moment. I know that they have quite a few characteristics that are different and that one seems to be confined to the glands and the other to the stromal cells, and this is something we obviously want to find out, what their different roles are.

5

Evaluation of menstrual blood loss – value of history and subjective assessment

M.P. Lamb

The most important evidence that a menstrual disorder is present is given in the history. A woman who has menstruated for years and then tells her doctor that the periods are getting heavier is either correct or her perception of increased loss is modified by other factors such as emotional upset, marital problems or a fear of genital cancer. An important fact is that the patient may complain of a change of menstrual pattern or increased heaviness. As most women would not generally wish for a gynaecological examination without reason it is commonly assumed that the complaint is genuine. Although her complaint may be genuine her assessment of the heaviness of her periods may not be very accurate.

The acceptance of menstrual loss is clearly and closely related to the individual approach to physiological processes and the psychological make-up of the individual patient. The changing status of women in society leads to an altered acceptance of menstrual symptoms[1].

HISTORY

Sudden change in menstrual loss is likely to be pathological and the development of clotting with particularly large well defined clots and pain with their passage ('clot colic') is a sign likely to suggest increased blood loss as the fibrinolytic system is overcome[2].

Some women confuse duration of menstruation with heaviness of menstrual flow[3] and although it has been shown that women with longer menstrual periods have a heavier loss Haynes and colleagues[4] in a study of 50 women in 1977 showed convincingly that there was no relation between the duration of menstruation and the total menstrual blood loss as 92% of the total menses were lost in the first 3 days. Fraser *et al.*[5] also showed that only 13% of their patients with menorrhagia has a flow for longer than 7 days, and Chimbira *et al.*[6] in a study with much greater numbers showed that only 11% had menstruation lasting more than 7 days.

A spontaneous retrospective assessment of heaviness of blood loss is commonly given in the history as a series of facts such as flooding, frequent soiling of under clothes, soiling of the bed and embarrassment. Ruined holidays or social mishaps, the need to use pads as well as tampons and the onset of tiredness and lethargy suggestive of the physical effects of anaemia, are frequent complaints. These historical extremes are often genuine and if not would be features of significant psychological or emotional disturbance. Menstrual changes in mental disturbance are not specific for any particular disease or syndrome but due as much to the secondary emotional upset as to the illness itself[7]. Younger women appear to be less tolerant of increasing menstrual loss than older women and would therefore assess periods as heavier for a given blood loss[5]. This is most likely related to the changing status of women in society which was alluded to earlier[1].

Symptoms of tiredness and lethargy, and rarely more serious physical effects of anaemia such as dyspnoea, may present in the history. Significant anaemia may occur with increasing menstrual loss as illustrated in a study of serum ferritin and blood loss associated with intrauterine contraceptive devices[8]. Up to 25% of patients had iron deficiency anaemia after 1 year of intrauterine contraceptive device use and related menorrhagia. However, not all women with menorrhagia have anaemia and it is certainly not a diagnostic feature (unpublished observations).

The accepted definition of menorrhagia is a loss of more than 80 ml by measured blood loss and was originally suggested by Hallberg *et al.*, in a menstrual blood loss–population study in 1966[9]. In this study the 95th centile of the normal range was 76.4 ml but in 1984 Fraser suggested that 60 ml may be a more realistic upper limit. In his study 41% of patients with subjective menorrhagia had a loss of less than that amount[5].

In another study of patients complaining of menorrhagia with known pelvic disease, patients with fibroids had significant measured blood loss which correlated well with the history although this was not so for other disorders[10]. van Eijkeran *et al.*, also showed that only five out of 21 patients awaiting hysterectomy for persistent menorrhagia had a measured blood loss of greater than 80 ml[11].

In the evaluation of therapy measured blood loss is much more useful than a history of menorrhagia[12], although other clinical studies of menorrhagia treatment with danazol using a detailed prospective but subjective menstrual calendar have produced results which compare favourably with findings using measured blood loss alone[13,14].

SUBJECTIVE ASSESSMENT

A prospective approach is much more likely to be accurate than the retrospective history. The menstrual calendar (Figure 1) has been used frequently and is simply a means by which the patient can record prospectively the features of her menstrual cycle.

The number of days bleeding are recorded as are the numbers of pads and tampons. The heaviness of the bleeding can be recorded on a scale from light to flooding. By using all the parameters of the assessment an evaluation of the blood loss can be made.

A method of interpreting the heaviness of the blood loss is by using a cumulative daily score and as a means of illustration details have been extracted from a trial assessing the effect of danazol and placebo on menstrual loss[14].

Heaviness

Patients were asked to rate the heaviness of their periods every day during the trial. However, rather than analyse each day separately the data was handled in the following way. For each rating the following score was awarded:
(1) less than normal,
(2) normal,

(3) heavy,
(4) very heavy,
(5) flooding.

These scores were totalled for each month of the trial to give an overall view of the heaviness of the period for each month. This method has some drawbacks in that the new scores have no real meaning in the way that the scores of 1–5 originally had. Also a numerical quantity has been placed on the variable so that, for example, a women who on 2 days rates her periods as normal then heavy has the same score as a women who on 1 day rates her period as flooding.

However, analysing each day separately would present us with the problem of repeating a statistical test many times where randomness could give significant results. This method does present us with a profile for heaviness for each patient and is more abstract than a visual analogue scale.

Pads and tampons

Pad and tampon counting has been helpful in showing a therapeutic response[14,15]. Other studies have shown no significance in the use of this

---

MENSTRUAL CALENDAR
Date of start of period _____

Days of your period		1 2 3 4 5 6 7 8 9 10 11 12 13 14
Heaviness of period		
Number of pads and tampons used	P	
	T	

Comments
Key
Flooding = A, very heavy = B, heavy = C, moderate = D, light = E.

Figure 1 Menstrual calendar for patients to record the features of their menstrual cycles. These can be of value in prospectively assessing subjective blood loss in subjects presenting with a history of presumed menorrhagia

MENSTRUAL CALENDAR
Date of start of period _____

Days of your period		1	2	3	4	5	6	7	8	9	10	11	12	13	14
Heaviness of period		D	B	A	A	B	C	E							
Number of pads and tampons used	P	2	9	12	10	8	5	1							
	T	6	9	10	14	8	5	2							

Comments
Key
Flooding = A, very heavy = B, heavy = C, moderate = D, light = E.

Excessive Menstrual Loss

MENSTRUAL CALENDAR
Date of start of period _____

Days of your period		1	2	3	4	5	6	7	8	9	10	11	12	13	14
Heaviness of period		E	C	C	D	D	E								
Number of pads and tampons used	P	0	3	4	0	0	0								
	T	4	10	11	8	7	3								

Comments
Key
Flooding = A, very heavy = B, heavy = C, moderate = D, light = E.

Moderate Menstrual Loss

Figure 1 *Continued from previous page*

assessment and in Fraser's study many of the women used large numbers of pads and tampons although some of the pads were barely discoloured after use[5]. Also it appears that the perception of volume might be based partly on the loss of other genital fluids not measured by a method based on detection of haemoglobin. The percentage contribution of blood to the total menstrual loss varies greatly with a mean of 36%[5].

The number of pads and tampons a woman uses will naturally depend on her personality. Other factors such as education, race, hygiene and social circumstances will have an important bearing on the rate of use. Therefore strictly as a measure of blood loss it must be regarded as unreliable but in the overall management of the patient it cannot be ignored.

Duration of bleeding

The number of days of bleeding is a simple fact recorded on the menstrual calendar but as mentioned earlier may not reliably reflect the amount of blood lost as most is lost in the first 3 days[4]. Prolonged bleeding however can be of major importance to the patient and in some instances will reflect a heavier loss[3].

CONCLUSION

A patient referred with heavy periods may give a good retrospective history of her blood loss but this is very unreliable as a true assessment of her menstrual loss and will only indicate that there is something wrong.

A subjective prospective assessment should be made and is likely to be a more reliable guide of her menstrual loss. A negative result, after the exclusion of disease may reassure the patient effectively and no further treatment may be required. If however the assessment is positive this could either be used as a guide to therapy or lead to further objective assessment before treatment.

Nevertheless patients with a change in menstrual loss even below the 80 ml criterion may find the increased bleeding unacceptable and wish for treatment. Reassurance after the exclusion of disease may not always satisfy. Empirical treatment should be considered or she may continue her pursuit elsewhere.

REFERENCES

1. Fisher, A.M. (1981). "Tis the hand of Nature and we women cannot escape it." *Clin. Obstet. Gynecol.*, **8**, 121–9
2. Skjodt, P. and Albrechtsen, O.K. (1965). Coagulation and fibrinolysis in uterine blood. *Acta Obstet. Gynaecol. Scand.*, **44**, 416–36
3. World Health Organization (1979). Special Programme of Research, Development and Research Training in Human Reproduction. *Eighth Annual Report*, 9.1. (Geneva: WHO)
4. Haynes, P.J., Hodgson, H. Anderson, A.B. and Turnbull, A.C. (1977). Measurement of menstrual blood loss in patients complaining of menorrhagia. *Br. J. Obstet. Gynaecol.*, **84**, 763–8
5. Fraser, I.S., McCarron, G. and Marram, R. (1984). A preliminary Study of factors influencing perception of menstrual blood loss volume. *Am. J. Obstet. Gynecol.*, **149**, 788–93
6. Chimbira, T.H., Anderson, A.B. and Turnbull, A.C. (1980). Relation between measured menstrual blood loss and patients subjective assessment of loss, duration of bleeding, number of sanitary towels used, uterine weight and endometrial surface area. *Br. J. Obstet. Gynaecol.*, **87**, 603–9
7. Carney, M.W.P. (1981). Menstrual disturbance: a psychogenic disorder? *Clin. Obstet. Gynecol.*, **8**, 103–9
8. Guillebaud, J., Barnett, M.D. and Gordon, Y.B. (1979). Plasma ferritin levels as an index of iron deficiency in women using intrauterine devices. *Br. J. Obstet. Gynaecol.*, **86**, 51–5
9. Hallberg, L., Hogdahl, A.M., Nilsson, L. and Rybo, G. (1966). Menstrual blood loss – a Population Study. *Acta Obstet. Gynaecol. Scand.*, **45**, 320
10. Fraser, I.S., McCarron, G., Markham, R., Resta, T. and Watts, A. (1986). Measured menstrual blood loss in women with menorrhagia associated with pelvic disease and coagulation disorder. *Obstet. Gynecol.*, **68**, 630–5
11. van-Eijkeran, M.A., Scholten, P.C., Christiaens, G.C., Alsbach, G. and Haspels, A.A. (1986). The alkaline haematin method for measuring menstrual blood loss a modification and its clinical use in menorrhagia. *Eur. J. Obstet. Gynaecol. Reprod. Biol.*, **22**, 345–51
12. Vasilenko, P., Kraicer, P.F., Kaplan, R., deMasi, A. and Freed, N. (1988). A new simple method of measuring menstrual blood loss. *J. Reprod. Med.*, **33**, 293–7
13. Fraser, I.S. (1985). Treatment of dysfunctional uterine bleeding with danazol. *Aust. N. Z. J. Obstet. Gynaecol.*, **25**, 224–6
14. Lamb, M.P. (1987). Danazol in menorrhagia; a double blind placebo controlled trial. *J. Obstet. Gynecol.*, **7**, 212–6
15. Jacubowcz, D.L. and Wood, C. (1979). The use of prostaglandin

synthetase inhibitor mefanemic acid in the treatment of menorrhagia. *Aust. N. Z. J. Obstet. Gynaecol.*, **18**, 135

DISCUSSION

Prof. I.S. Fraser   I feel strongly that we should have a short discussion on definitions. Dr Lamb has raised one aspect of that in mentioning a comment that I made in a paper that perhaps 60 ml was a more realistic cut-off than 80 ml for menorrhagia. Either is arbitrary, but in the original Hallberg, Nilsson and Rybo study all the haematological parameters begin to drop in the group that are regularly losing blood at >60 ml per cycle. I would also be interested for people to make their comments on what they feel dysfunctional uterine bleeding is and what their own definitions of that are. Very few papers define it, very few textbooks define it, and in different countries people mean totally different things by the terminology.

Dr J.M. Higham   Again it is whether it is a problem to the woman to a certain extent. I see a number of women who are chronically anaemic for no apparent cause who consider their menstruation to be normal and I find it to be excessive. Recently I looked at 100 of my women and I did a comparison between their baseline haemoglobin and their subsequent menstrual blood loss. There is a wide scatter in that data but there was a negative correlation of about 0.5.

Mr M.P. Lamb   Dysfunctional uterine bleeding as far as I am concerned is a clinical diagnosis. The patient who complains that she cannot stand her periods any longer has a problem and we then have to try to quantify what that problem is. If we exclude disease, then we have to say she has dysfunctional uterine bleeding. Whether she can be treated by simple reassurance or simple drug therapy, or requires a hysterectomy, or an endometrial ablation is a matter of decision afterwards.

Prof. R.W. Shaw   We are really trying to address the problem of what is presumed excessive menstrual period blood loss; not total blood loss which may be erratic throughout the cycle, but heavy or prolonged menstrual periods on a regular cyclic basis in the absence of any endocrine or haematological disorder which would explain it, and in the absence of any gross pathology of the uterus (fibroids, adenomyosis).

Prof. I.S. Fraser That is actually very important – whether we just exclude gross pelvic pathology. Quite a number of studies have now shown that 40% of patients who initially on reasonable clinical examination, including applying curettage, are given a diagnosis of dysfunctional uterine bleeding, will be shown to have organic pathology which could have accounted for their symptoms.

I would make a plea for the progressive introduction of out-patient hysteroscopy with the new flexible fibre optic hysteroscopes and directed biopsy rather than blind curettage that we have been doing for years and missing a lot of pathology. That is critical if we shall be moving to endometrial ablations – where current experts are finding all sorts of pathology in patients referred to them of which they were unaware after blind curettage.

Dr M.C.P. Rees I am interested in the psychological aspects of the complaint of menorrhagia. Studies done in Oxford over the past 10 years show no psychological differences between women complaining of menorrhagia and those not complaining of menorrhagia, whether or not the menorrhagia exists.

Mr M.P. Lamb I was not suggesting that there is anything necessarily wrong with these women, but if they are complaining and they do not have problems then that would suggest that there is some major emotional or psychological background such as a marital problem.

6

Measured menstrual blood losses – normal population and 'menorrhagic' patients

J.M. Higham and R.W. Shaw

The need to quantify menstrual loss objectively has previously been emphasized, owing to the unreliability of history taking and other subjective assessments[1]. Previous authors have commented that the complaint of excessive bleeding, the use of a high number of sanitary towels and tampons per period and the duration of the menses are not necessarily correlated with objective menorrhagia[2-4]. Clinical examination which revealed the presence of a bulky uterus has previously been considered responsible for higher menstrual blood losses[5]. However, data from 100 patients attending the Royal Free Hospital demonstrated no significant correlation between the ultrasonically measured estimate of uterine volume and menstrual blood loss (Figure 1). Similarly, the degree to which the endometrium was thickened in the mid-luteal phase was not predictive of subsequent loss (Figure 2). This lack of correlation was the same for both parous and nulliparous women. These findings agree with those of Chimbira *et al.*[1] who measured the uterine weight and endometrial surface area (also hypothesized as relating to menstrual blood loss[6]) of 40 women at the time of hysterectomy. Having estimated their menstrual loss prior to the operation, they also could not confirm an association between these parameters and the quantity of blood lost.

The lack of reliable predictors as to the amount of blood lost by an individual at the time of menstruation means it has been necessary to

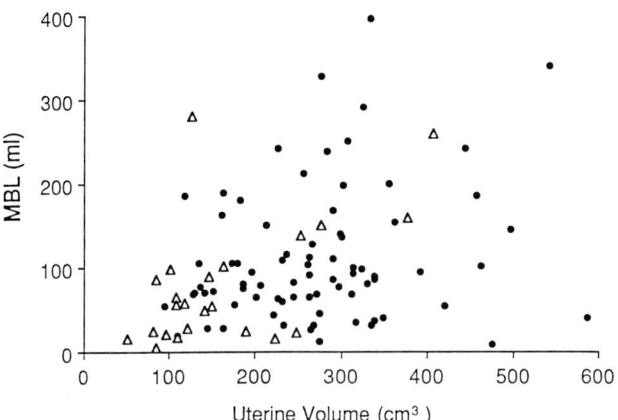

Figure 1 Correlation between uterine volume, estimated ultrasonically, and menstrual blood loss (MBL) in parous (●) and nulliparous (Δ) women; $n=100$, $r=0.329$

assay this volume. A variety of techniques have been developed over the years to achieve this. These can be divided into four main method groupings, but this listing is not exhaustive. In 1964 Göltner and Gailer described a technique whereby they measured the electrical conductivity of the solution resulting from the immersion of used sanitary towels in water[7]. The electrolyte concentration (and hence conductivity) of the fluid being proportional to the blood volume present. The remaining methods to be described can be divided into the following main groupings:

(1) weight estimates,
(2) radioisotope methods,
(3) iron determination, and
(4) haemoglobin determination.

WEIGHT ESTIMATES

The weighing of soiled sanitary material as a means of menstrual blood loss assessment was described some 90 years ago in a thesis by Prussag[8]. This method was again used by Pendergrass *et al.* who provided standardsets of preweighed sanitary supplies which were then reweighed following the menses[9]. As every item both used and unused was returned,

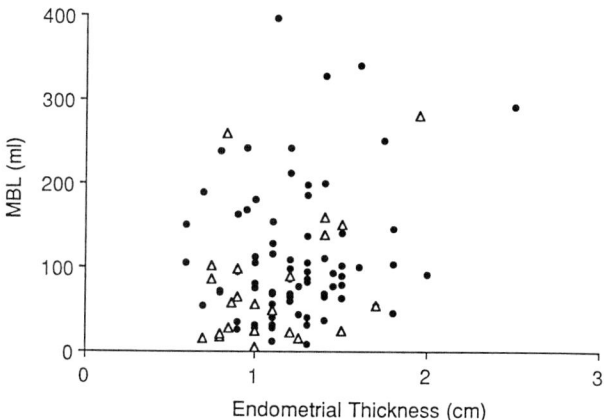

Figure 2 Correlation between endometrial thickness at the mid-luteal phase and menstrual blood loss (MBL), in parous (●) and nulliparous (Δ) women; $n=100$, $r=0.185$

the additional weight postmenses was assumed to be due to absorbed menstrual fluid. This simple technique of weighing however, estimates only the total menstrual loss and is not specific for blood. The contribution of blood to menstrual fluid has been shown to vary considerably, Fraser quoted figures ranging between 1.6% and 82%[10]. This factor, combined with other potential errors introduced by contamination of the collection with other substances such as urine and variable evaporation, results in the method having limited usefulness.

The remaining techniques are more specifically directed towards the blood component of menstrual loss.

RADIOISOTOPE METHODS

Radioisotopic markers have been employed, for example iron (^{59}Fe)[11] and chromium (^{51}Cr)[12-14]. These isotopes have been used to label red blood cells premenstrually, the activity in the peripheral circulation being measured at the commencement and cessation of the menses. During menstruation all used towels and tampons are collected, and the level of activity of this collection is assessed. The quantity of menstrual blood lost can then be calculated from the scintillation counts of the collection and the mean of the two venous blood estimates.

71

Similar premenses red cell labelling with ^{59}Fe has been combined with the counting of whole body radioactivity[15,16]. The fall in the level of radioactivity measured postmenstrually is proportional to the quantity of blood that is lost. It was hoped that this technique would overcome the need to collect used sanitary material (such collections frequently being incomplete, secondary to unavoidable blood loss occurring at such times as visits to the lavatory). Unfortunately however, this technique was found to lack sufficient accuracy when estimating blood losses in the normal range. Price *et al.* quoted inaccuracies of between 20 and 40 ml per period as not being unusual[15]. Holt felt that the method was only sensitive enough to detect blood loss in the order of 100–300 ml, and then with limited accuracy and suggested it should be used clinically when the blood loss concerned was above 700 ml[16]. In addition, the method is not specific to menstrual blood, bleeding from other sites (for example for peptic ulceration) would contribute to an over-estimation of menstrual blood loss. Finally, concerning all the radioisotopic methods, on occasion there is reticence to administer and to receive these compounds, even though the dosages of radioactivity are small.

IRON DETERMINATION

The iron content of sanitary towels and tampons is proportional to the blood retained within them and can be estimated by a variety of techniques[17]. Thomas described wet oxidation and dry-ashing procedures of chemical iron determination[17]. These methods are both sensitive and accurate but are also time consuming involving many steps when performing the assay. A more rapid measurement of iron content using atomic absorption spectrophotometry, enables the omission of several steps in the preparation of samples[18]. Cheyne and Shepherd demonstrated this method to give results sufficiently close to those using the chemical method to validate its use[19].

HAEMOGLOBIN DETERMINATION

The haemoglobin content of menstrual collections has also been used to estimate menstrual blood loss. Haemoglobin is converted to a coloured, haematin compound in either acid[20] or alkaline[21] solution. This colorimetric method, described by Hallberg and Nilsson in 1964[21], is currently the most widely used and it is a reliable technique of assessing menstrual blood loss. The optical density of the solution resulting from incubation of used sanitary towels and tampons in 5% aqueous sodium hydroxide can be measured with a spectrophotometer. If a sample of venous blood is incubated in parallel to the menstrual collection, it is possible to calculate the volume of menstrual blood. Modifications to the method have subsequently been published[22], but the basic principle remains the same. The method has been validated[23,24], Rees and colleagues quoting a recovery *in vitro* of 95 ± 5% with intra- and interassay coefficients of variation of 8% and 9% respectively[24]. This manual method requires an incubation period of 48 hours for the colour intensity to stabilize. Extensive squeezing and massaging of the sanitary material is also needed to ensure the complete elution and conversion of the haemoglobin. Such a delay and need for manual effort is overcome using a mechanical device as described by Newton in 1977[25]. The use of such an automatic extractor enables a reading to be taken after only 15 minutes of mechanical pummelling.

Methods such as those described above have enabled quantification of menstrual loss in the population. Three of the larger studies measuring menstrual blood loss are summarized in Table 1. There have been many other studies performed but the numbers of women concerned were small. Of the studies listed in Table 1 a variety of the techniques for blood quantification were used. Barer and Fowler determined the iron content following chemical digestion in collections made by 100 healthy women, the majority of whom were hospital workers[3]. Cole measured the iron by atomic absorption spectrophotometry in a study of the menstruating female population of a Northumberland mining village[6]. Finally, Hallberg and his colleagues used the alkaline haemtin technique, which they had published 2 years previously, when considering a group of 476 women resident in the town of Göteborg in Sweden[2]. These studies show menstrual blood loss to have a positive skew distribution. The figure of approximately 80 ml represents the 95th centile of the distribution and losses above this are regarded as pathological.

The perception however, of what should be considered a normal menses varies widely. For example, in a group of 151 women who

Table 1 Population studies of menstrual blood loss (ml) per menses; n=number of women

	n	*Range*	*Mean*	*Median*
Barer & Fowler[3]	100	6.6–178.7	50.6	35.9
Hallberg *et al.*[2]	476	—	43.4	30.0
	(137)	(1.6–200)		
Cole *et al.*[6]	348	0.1–280	37.5	27.5

complained of excessively heavy periods only 57% were found to have a loss in excess of 80 ml when quantified by the alkaline haematin method. Losses in this group ranged from 10.2 to 635.8 ml with a median value of 94 ml. Similarly, 48 women who considered themselves to have menses of completely normal quantity had blood losses which were between 1.4 to 288 ml when objectively quantified (median 38.6 ml) (Figure 3).

This is comparable with the work carried out by Chimbira *et al.* who asked women to assess their periods as being either light, moderate or heavy and found a large overlap in measured menstrual losses between all three groups of women, similar to our findings shown in Figure 3. The inability to rely upon an assessment by any individual as to the amount of her loss has been repeatedly commented upon[2,4,12]. Fraser *et al.* found when measuring blood loss as part of a drug trial for menorrhagia that only 38% of the women had a loss in excess of 80 ml[4].

In an attempt to increase the accuracy of menstrual blood loss quantification, with a method which does not require the use of laboratory facilities, a pictorial blood loss assessment chart (PBAC) was devised (Figure 4). It has been previously noted[12] that simple inspection of soiled sanitary material gives a reasonably accurate assessment of its blood contents, and it has been remarked that many sanitary items were only slightly soiled with blood.

The PBAC consisted of diagrams representing lightly, moderately and heavily soiled sanitary towels and tampons. The passage of clots and episodes of flooding were also noted. A PBAC was given to patients together with an instruction leaflet and standard sanitary supplies (Kotex size 2 towels/super plus tampons). The chart was completed at the same time as the used sanitary items were collected and both were returned to the laboratory. This collection was then subjected to a similar assessment

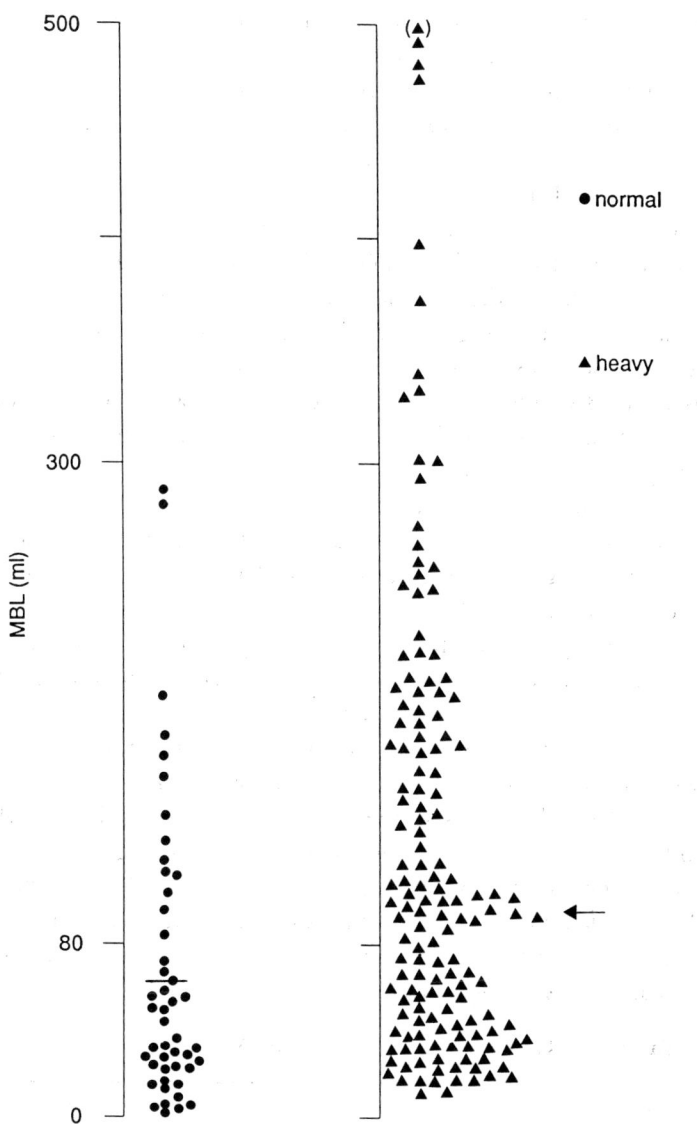

Figure 3 Scatter plots of menstrual blood loss in women who considered their loss to be normal (●; *n*=48, range 1.4–288 ml) and those who considered it to be excessively heavy (Δ; *n*=151, range 10.2–635.8 ml)

by a single gynaecologist employing a PBAC. Finally, the blood content of each menstrual collection was determined by the alkaline haematin technique[21]. Ascending scores were awarded for increasingly blood stained sanitary towels/tampons and the total obtained from each chart was compared with the blood loss in ml for that cycle. Statistical analysis was performed using Spearman Rank correlation coefficients. The results are presented in Table 2.

A close correlation ($r=0.847$) was found between the 55 patient PBAC scores and menstrual blood loss (Figure 5). Similarly, the 122 gynaecologist PBAC cycle scores, demonstrated a close correlation ($r=0.872$) with menstrual blood loss (Figure 6). The patient and gynaecologist PBAC scores were also shown to correlate well ($r=0.899$) (Figure 7).

Taking a PBAC score of 100 or more as a diagnostic test of menorrhagia gave a sensitivity of 86% and a specificity of 89%, using the patients' scores. (These figures were 86% and 81% respectively for the gynaecologist.)

The reliability of this method of menstrual blood loss assessment is increased by the fact that standard sanitary towels/tampons were supplied, it having been previously noted that the absorption capacity of such items can vary greatly[26].

It is interesting to note that women do appear to have a quite accurate perception as to how heavily items are soiled; a factor important for the use of such a chart. Having demonstrated a close correlation between menstrual blood loss and the PBAC scoring, this chart represents a new simple method of assessment. This could be useful in almost any clinical situation where it would be desirable to assess the complaint of menorrhagia, which is currently rarely substantiated before either medical or surgical treatment[27].

As has been previously demonstrated in this paper, menorrhgia may well be complained of in the presence of a completely normal blood loss. This chart may assist in reassurance of such women, thus avoiding unnecessary intervention.

Table 2 Results obtained using the PBAC

	Range	Median
Patient PBAC scores	5–456	121
Gynaecologist PBAC scores	6–630	87
Menstrual blood loss (ml)	1.9–366.4	73.8

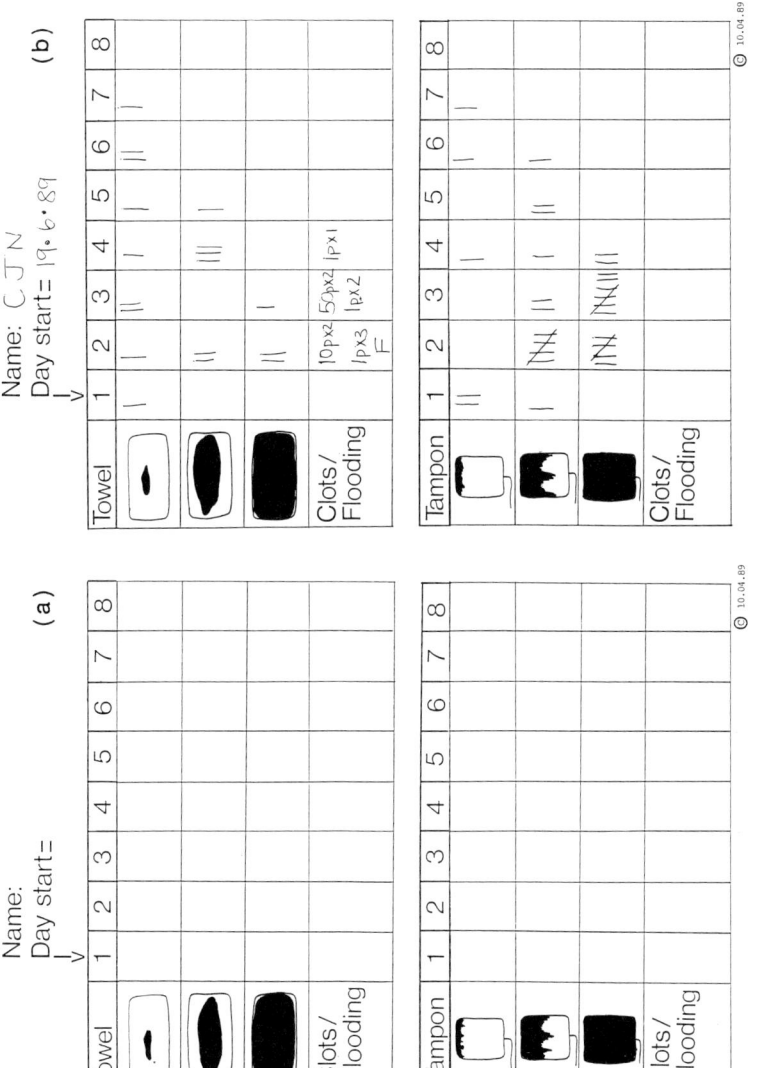

Figure 4 PBAC (a) and PBAC filled in by a menorrhagic patient (b)

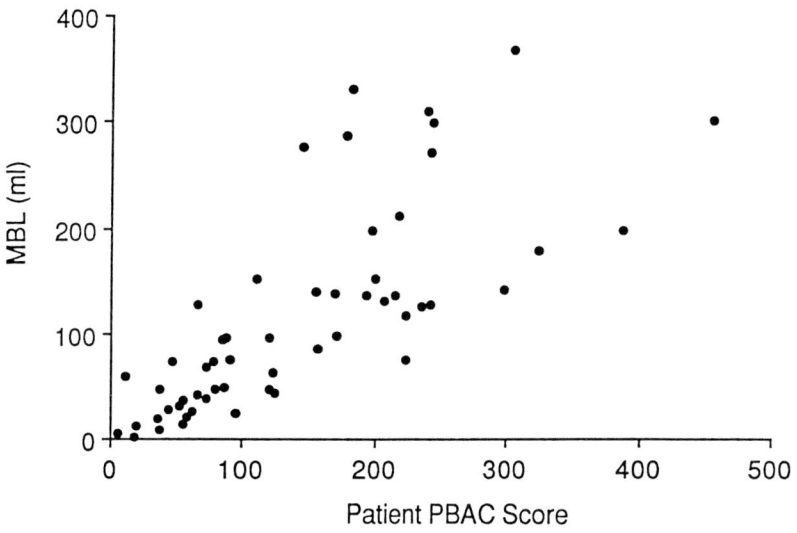

Figure 5 Correlation between patient PBAC score and menstrual blood loss (MBL); *n*=55, *r*=0.847

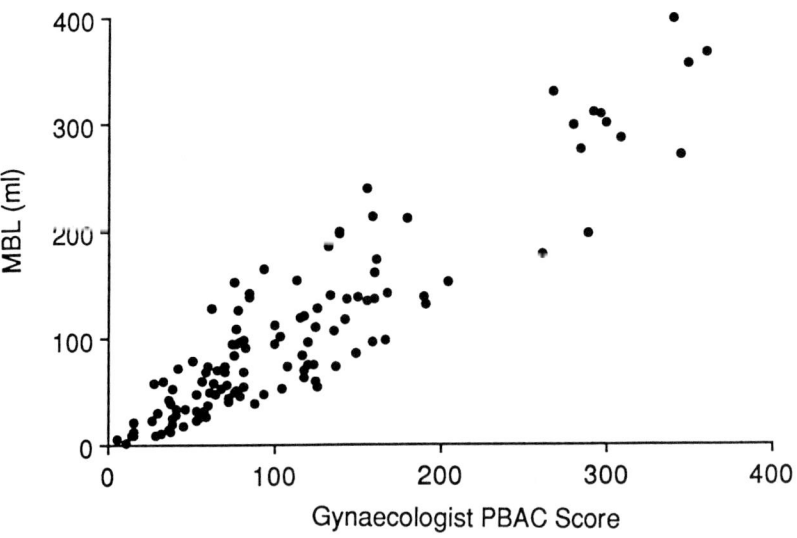

Figure 6 Correlation between gynaecologist PBAC score and menstrual blood loss (MBL); *n*=122, *r*=0.872

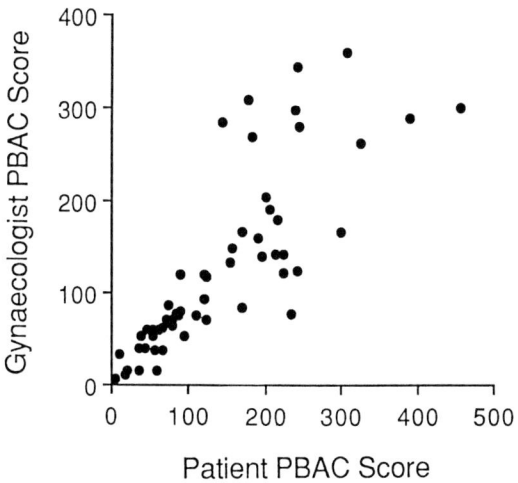

Figure 7   Correlation between gynaecologist and patient PBAC scores; $n=55$, $r=0.899$

ACKNOWLEDGEMENTS

We are most grateful to Professor P.M.S. O'Brien for his invaluable assistance in the conception and design of the PBAC.

We also thank E. Naylor for the German translation, and Winthrop Labs for the sponsorship of J. Higham.

REFERENCES

1. Chimbira, T.H., Anderson, A.B.M. and Turnbull, A.C. (1980). Relation between measured menstrual blood loss and patient's subjective assessment of loss, duration of bleeding, number of sanitary towels used, uterine weight and endometrial surface area. *Br. J. Obstet. Gynaecol.*, **87**, 603–9

2. Hallberg, L., Hogdahl, A., Nilsson, L. and Rybo, G. (1966). Menstrual blood loss – a population study. *Acta Obstet. Gynecol. Scand.*, **45**, 320–51

3. Barer, A.P. and Fowler, W.M. (1936). The blood loss during normal menstruation. *Am. J. Obstet. Gynecol.*, **31**, 979–86

4. Fraser, I.S., McCarron, G. and Markham, R. (1984). A preliminary study of factors influencing perception of menstrual blood loss volume. *Am. J. Obstet. Gynecol.*, **149**, 788–93

5. Honore, L.H. (1979). Menorrhagia, diffuse myometrial hypertrophy and

the intrauterine contraceptive device: a report of fourteen cases. *Acta Obstet. Gynecol. Scand.*, **58**, 283–5

6. Cole, S.K., Billewicz, W.Z. and Thomson, A.M. (1971). Sources of variation in menstrual blood loss. *J. Obstet. Gynaecol. Br. Cwlth.*, **78**, 933–9

7. Goltner, E. and Gailer, H.J. (1964). Blutverlust bei der Menstruation. *Zentralbl. Gynakol.*, **86**, 1177–87

8. Prussag. St. Petersburg thesis, cited in reference 12.

9. Pendergrass, P.B., Scott, J.N. and Ream, L.J. (1984). A rapid, noninvasive method for evaluation of total menstrual loss. *Gynecol. Obstet. Invest.*, **17**, 174–8

10. Fraser, I.S., McCarron, G., Markham, R. and Resta, T. (1985). Blood and total fluid content of menstrual discharge. *Obstet. Gynecol.*, **65**, 194–8

11. Baldwin, R.M., Whalley, P.J. and Pritchard, J.A. (1961). Measurements of menstrual blood loss. *Am. J. Obstet. Gynecol.*, **81**, 739–42

12. Rankin, G.L.S., Veall, N., Huntsman, R.G. and Liddell, J. (1962). Measurement with 51 Cr of red-cell loss in menorrhagia. *Lancet*, **1**, 567–9

13. Jacobs, A. and Butler, E.B. (1965). Menstrual blood-loss in iron-deficiency anaemia. *Lancet*, **2**, 407–9

14. Tauxe, W.N. (1962). Quantitation of menstrual blood loss: a radioactive method utilizing a counting dome. *J. Nucl. Med.*, **3**, 282–7

15. Price, D.C., Forsyth, E.M., Cohn, S.H. and Cronkite, E.P. (1964). The study of menstrual and other blood loss, and consequent iron deficiency, by Fe 59 whole-body counting. *J. Assoc. Med. Canad.*, **90**, 51–4

16. Holt, J.M., Mayet, F.G.H., Warner, G.T. and Callender, S.T. (1967). Measurement of blood loss by means of a whole-body counter. *Br. Med. J.*, **4**, 86–8

17. Thomas, J.D.R. (1969). The determination of menstrual iron loss. *Biochem. Med.*, **3**, 311–20

18. Hefnawi, F., Saleh, A.A., Kandil, O. and Yacout, M.M. (1975). Blood loss with IUCDs. In Hefnawi, F. and Segal, S.J. (eds). *Analysis of Intrauterine Contraception*, pp. 373–80 (New York: American Elsevier Publishing Co.)

19. Cheyne, G.A. and Shepherd, M.M. (1970). Comparison of chemical and atomic absorption methods for estimating menstrual blood loss. *J. med. Lab. Technol.*, **27**, 350–4

20. Hoppe-Seyler, G. and Brodensen, R. (1904). Ueber den Blutverlust bei der Menstruation. *Z. Physiol. Chem.*, **42**, 545–53

21. Hallberg, L. and Nilsson, L. (1964). Determination of menstrual blood loss. *Scand. J. Lab. Invest.*, **16**, 244–8

22. van Eijkeren, M.A., Scholten, P.C., Christiaens, C.M.L., Alsbach, G.P.J. and Haspels, A.A. (1986). The alkaline haematin method for measuring menstrual blood loss – a modification and its clinical use in menorrhagia.

Eur. J. Obstet. Gynaecol. Reprod. Biol., **22**, 345–51

23. Rees, M.C.P., Chimbira, T.H., Anderson, A.B.M. and Turnbull, A.C. (1982). Menstrual blood loss: measurement and clinical correlates. *Res. Clin. Forums*, **4**, 69–80

24. Shaw, S.T., Aaronson, D.E. and Moyer, D.L. (1972). Quantitation of menstrual blood loss - further evaluation of the alkaline hematin method. *Contraception*, **5**, 497–513

25. Newton, J., Barnard, G. and Collins, W. (1977). A rapid method for measuring menstrual blood loss using automatic extraction. *Contraception*, **16**, 269–82

26. Grimes, D.A. (1979). Estimating vaginal blood loss. *J. Reprod. Med.*, **22**, 190–2

27. Smith, S.K. (1988). Mechanisms and management of dysmenorrhoea and menorrhagia – a reassessment. *Br. J. Sex. Med.*, July

DISCUSSION

Dr M.A. Lumsden   Women when they come to the out-patients are not complaining of heavy menstrual blood loss. They are complaining of heavy menstrual fluid loss. It is known that blood is a variable proportion of menstrual fluid, and sometimes I think we try to change the menstrual blood loss when so many of the women are not actually anaemic.

It is possible that menstrual fluid may contain a lot of factors which may be contributing to the tiredness, the depression, etc. which so often goes with menstruation. Maybe we should spend more time on trying to assess a little bit more about the fluid than simply the blood. Clotting apart, obviously.

Dr J.M. Higham   I would thoroughly agree. A lot of women say that they are not actually passing blood, 'just that watery stuff'. That is equally inconvenient for them and we should perhaps do more studies to measure the quantity of fluid that women lose by that simple weighing technique.

Prof. I S. Fraser   It is a real thorny question assessing menstrual loss. The system that Dr Higham has described (Patient Blood Loss Assessment Chart – PBAC) with more refinement could almost certainly be made even more accurate. It is already more accurate than I have been able to make my own clinical assessment, blind at the first time I see the patient, by asking leading questions based on our previous studies. But there are quite a number of problems that lead to errors within such a system.

We find that a proportion of the women who have a complaint of menorrhagia which is not substantiated on measurement on close questioning, are losing blood in gushes much more than a fairly steady loss and that the blood is flowing round the pad or tampon quite quickly and is staining their underclothes, flooding in the bed, etc.

Dr H. Critchley When assessing a patient who is complaining of menorrhagia, what is the intra–patient variation in menstrual blood loss from cycle to cycle? Is it fairly constant so that on assessing one or two cycles a decision can be reached as to whether or not they do have menorrhagia?

Dr J.M. Higham There are two aspects to that question. Most women, even though they cannot tell whereabouts they are on the scale, can quite often tell differences between a heavy period and a light period and what is average for them and what is not.

There is a cyclicity to menstruation, but I would certainly feel confident that there is not that much variation between one period and another, and if one woman comes in with a large collection, on the whole I have not seen a dramatic fall with other collections.

Mr E. Versi If we were to take a cut off of 60–80 ml, because that is what results in changes in haematological indices, that is correct if we are to treat the haematological problem. But there will still be patients who have blood loss that is less than that for whom it is a problem. Is it that these patients are experiencing change in their menstrual loss in that they have had an increased loss, and if that is the case how can we look at that formally?

Dr J.M. Higham My study was of a fairly heterogeneous group of women and one cannot make global statements for them all.

If we are talking about assessment of change, a typical change occurs for example when a woman stops the pill and gets a return of her 'normal' menstruation. For that type of group we would be likely to gain some reassurance. It is to go beyond that and prove that a woman does not suffer from menorrhagia, but she still feels that she has a problem. Ethically should we or should we not give treatment?

Dr A.J. Gordon I remember in training being taught that women who use tampons alone do not have significant menorrhagia. From the pictorial studies is there any further information about women who are menorrhagic who use tampons alone and who do not use towels.

Dr J.M. Higham A lot of my women who are menorrhagic use exclusively tampons. They take them out at very frequent intervals and they are completely sodden with blood. I would not say that method, sanitary towel or tampon usage, was at all indicative.

Dr H.P. McEwan Perhaps one of the points arising from this meeting is the need to educate not only patients but also general practitioners, trying to educate them not to refer those women who probably do not have major problems.

Prof. R.W. Shaw I would agree. That would certainly reduce the pressure on gynaecological out-patients. But unless they can evaluate patients effectively they might miss patients who do need to be referred. Development of accurate subjective methods is thus essential to progress with this complaint.

7

Menorrhagia – the cost and scope of treatment

M. A. Lumsden

Menorrhagia, or excessive menstrual loss, causes considerable morbidity for women of reproductive age and is also a common cause of iron deficiency anaemia in the UK[1]. It is a problem which is increasing in importance; the National Morbidity Survey which collects data for general practice consultations in England and Wales suggests that between 1971 and 1981 the consultations for abnormal uterine bleeding have increased by 73%[2]. This may be due to the fact that women now experience more menstrual cycles, since many limit the size of their families and the duration of lactation. The morbidity and loss of efficiency which may occur as a result of a recurring problem such as menorrhagia is considerable and requires prompt, safe and effective treatment. This paper looks at the main types of therapy for menorrhagia and tries to assess their effectiveness as well as the cost to both the patient and the National Health Service (NHS). It will be concerned principally with dysfunctional uterine bleeding where there is no organic pathology within the uterus although I am sure most people are now aware that abnormal uterine function may still be present.

HYSTERECTOMY

Hysterectomy, the effectiveness of which cannot be disputed, is the traditional treatment for menstrual problems. There is very rarely any objective evaluation of the menstrual blood loss prior to operation despite the fact that the subjective and objective assessment of blood loss do not correlate[3]. Women are not good at assessing their own menstrual loss and only about half of those complaining of menorrhagia actually have a loss greater than 80 ml per menses[4,5] which is considered the upper limit of normal[6]. Patient satisfaction is an important aspect of evaluation since this operation is usually carried out to improve the quality of life, rather than as a life-saving procedure. Most British studies report high levels of satisfaction with the operation[7] although the physical morbidity of hysterectomy is high. When factors such as pyrexia, haemorrhage requiring transfusion and further unplanned surgery are considered then the incidence of side-effects may be as much as 43% for abdominal and 24% for vaginal hysterectomy[8]. There is also a significant mortality rate estimated in one American study of 437 000 women to be six per 10 000 in those not pregnant, without cancer and under 54 years old[9]. Psychological sequelae have also been the subject of study although it is often difficult to be sure that problems occurring are actually due to the operation itself. Another factor of considerable importance is that women perceive fluid rather than blood loss. Blood is a variable constituent of menstrual fluid and heavy fluid loss may not be a cause of anaemia, but may deplete other unknown factors as well as being immensely inconvenient. Fifty per cent of the uteri removed at hysterectomy are normal in structure and in these cases abnormal prostaglandin production is likely to be contributing to any increased blood loss[10]. Figures from the Oxford Family Planning Association study (which includes data from the private sector) suggests that 38% of the uteri removed from women under 45 years old have normal uterine histology[11].

It is a matter of debate as to whether these uteri should be removed or the problem treated by other means. Figures from the Scottish Home & Health Department showing the cost of hospital treatment of menorrhagia in rather more objective terms are shown in Table 1. In 1987 31 962 bed days were occupied with the primary complaint of menorrhagia, a majority taken by patients having a hysterectomy. Each bed day costs approximately £206 covering nursing costs, the running of the ward, etc. The cost of running an operating theatre is difficult to determine but in the private sector the surgeon/anaesthetist fees as described by BUPA are £590 and theatre charge £193 (1989).

Table 1 The number of operations and days spent overnight in hospital in Scotland by women with the primary indication of menorrhagia during the year 1987. Figures were obtained from the Information Services Division of the Scottish Health Service Common Services Agency

	No. of operations	*Bed days*
Total abdominal hysterectomy	2 300	22 437
Myomectomy	96	1 236
Dilatation & Curettage	3 831	4 755
Other operations	1 147	2 332
No operation	401	1 202
Total		31 962

The number of hysterectomies performed in the UK as a whole is gradually increasing[12] and figures for Scotland are shown in Figure 1. These figures are an underestimate since they do not include those performed in the private sector. Hysterectomy rates vary considerably between countries; 20% of women living in England and Wales will have a hysterectomy before the age of 65. This figure is 50% in California[13]. There is also a marked difference between different areas and social groups in many countries although this is less within the UK[14]. There are many factors which may explain this, including patterns of referral, gynaecological practice and patient expectation since there does not appear to be a regional variation in the problem itself. These factors may not be constant since a decrease in the numbers of hysterectomies in Ticino canton, Switzerland was achieved by a mass media campaign[15] which changed the attitudes of both gynaecologists and patients. This study suggests that unnecessary operations are being performed which is important when considering the problems already discussed and also that women spend about 10 days in hospital and many months recovering as a result of this procedure.

Hysterectomy may be performed by either the abdominal or vaginal route. The commonest reason for performing abdominal hysterectomy is the presence of leiomyomata (fibroids) and these are also a common cause of menorrhagia. Bleeding problems lead to many vaginal hysterectomies, although in many centres this procedure is rarely performed without a degree of prolapse. Dicker *et al.*[8] discussed the results of 1851

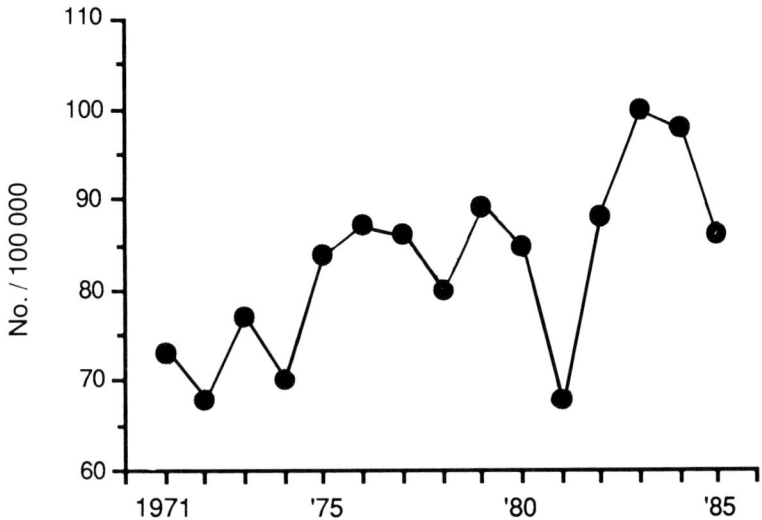

Figure 1 The number of hysterectomies per 100 000 women performed in Scotland between 1971 and 1985 (1981 was the year complicated by industrial action)

hysterectomies and found the incidence of febrile morbidity, haemorrhage requiring transfusion and readmission to hospital more common in women having abdominal hysterectomy. In the group of women who could have had their operation by either route 60 000 bed days could be saved each year in the USA by performing all hysterectomies by the vaginal route. Recent studies suggest that uterine enlargement due to the presence of fibroids may be reduced by the administration of a luteinizing hormone-releasing hormone (LHRH) agonist[16,17]. This could allow more to be performed by the vaginal route and it also has been found to facilitate the operation when the abdominal route is preferred[18]. Therefore pretreatment with LHRH agonists could reduce the cost of operation for both patient and the NHS.

MEDICAL TREATMENT

It is surprising that the number of hysterectomies for menorrhagia has not fallen as the number of medical treatments available has increased in recent years. The number of prescriptions written in the UK for the year up to

December 1988 is shown in Table 2. Norethisterone is the most popular but it is only very recently that it has been properly evaluated. Its use was probably based on the premise that menorrhagia was due to anovulation although this is now known to account for only about 20% of cases[19].

A recent, as yet unpublished, study[20], compares the efficacy of mefenamic acid with norethisterone. Both were similarly effective in reducing menstrual blood loss (Figure 2) although median loss was still above the upper limit of normal in both groups. It is well known that subjective assessment and objective measurement of blood loss do not correlate[3] and more women appeared satisfied with the mefenamic acid than the norethisterone (Table 3), although in nine of 17 women on mefenamic acid and eight of 15 women on norethisterone loss remained in excess of 80 ml. Minor side-effects occurred in 60–70% of women but only one subject in each group chose to discontinue treatment (Table 4).

This is an important point since the success of any treatment involves comparing the efficacy with the side-effects. A recent comparison between mefenamic acid and danazol[21] suggests that although side-effects

Table 2 The number of prescriptions written in the UK for drugs to treat menorrhagia during the year 1988. Figures quoted by kind permission of Warner Lambert Ltd (Total 626 000)

Name	Number of prescriptions
Norethisterone	204 000
Mefenamic acid	89 000
Danazol	63 000
Ethamsylate	70 000

Table 3 Patient satisfaction with norethisterone and mefenamic acid. Patients were asked to indicate their response on the scale: 1 = Good improvement; 2 = Some improvement; 3 = Unchanged; and 4 = Worse

	4	3	2	1
Norethisterone	3	3	6	3
Mefenamic acid	9	5	3	0

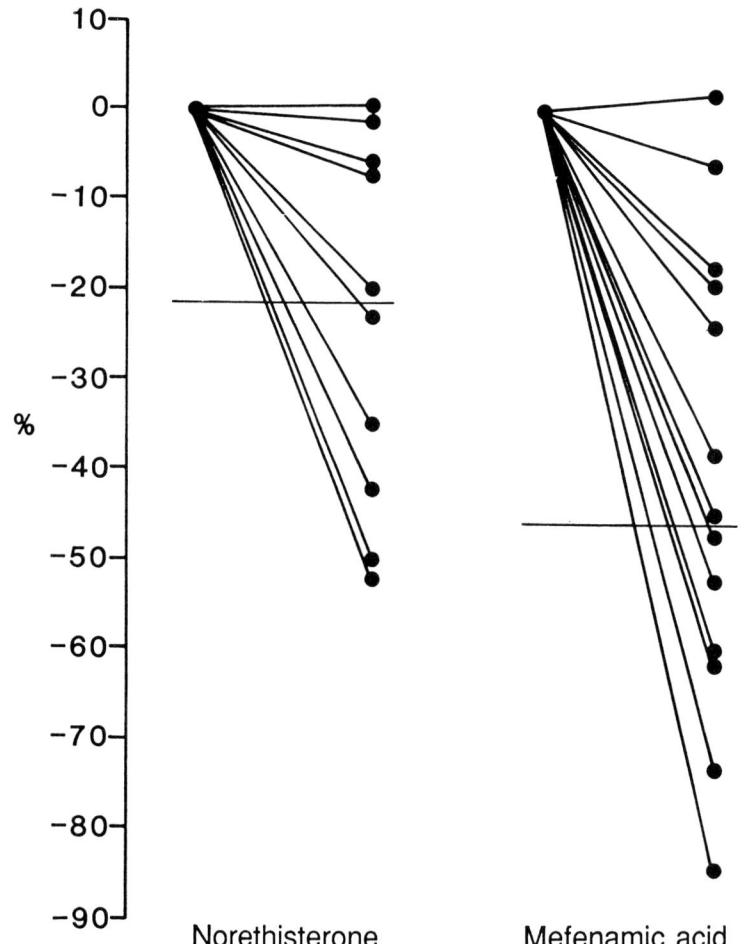

Figure 2 The percentage change in menstrual blood loss in women receiving Primolut™ (norethisterone) or Ponstan (mefenamic acid). The median is indicated by the bar

occurred in 75% of those on danazol and only 30% of those on mefenamic acid, similar numbers (50%) of women wished to continue the treatment at the end of the trial period since danazol produced a significantly greater decrease in the menstrual blood loss than mefenamic acid (60% as compared with 20%). However, danazol is normally only prescribed for a limited period of time since the metabolic and endocrinological effects of administering it over long periods of time are

Table 4 The side-effects experienced by the subjects taking norethisterone or mefenamic acid

	Mefenamic acid	*Norethisterone*
None	7 (41%)	4 (27%)
Headache	4 (24%)	5 (33%)
Abdominal pain	3 (18%)	3 (20%)
Nausea	2 (12%)	1 (7%)
Other	7 (41%)	6 (40%)

unknown and at the end of treatment the loss gradually increases to original levels[22].

The antifibrinolytic agents are also used in the treatment of menorrhagia. Epsilonamino-caproic acid and tranexamic acid reduce excessive menstrual blood loss by 47% and 54% respectively[23]. Side-effects are again common (50%) and include nausea, dizziness, diarrhoea, headache and abdominal pain. Intracranial thrombosis has been reported[24] since systemic fibrinolytic activity is slightly reduced. Ethamsylate, a drug which probably acts by reducing capillary fragility, also reduces the menstrual blood loss by round 50%[24].

The actual cost of treatment and the impact of side-effects on the patient will obviously be affected by the duration of treatment. Women may require medication for many years which gives drugs taken only during the menses a distinct advantage. Although mefenamic acid is only partially effective in reducing the menstrual blood loss it has the advantage of being taken for only 3–5 days each month. This makes it economical and also is likely to reduce the incidence of serious side-effects. This is true also of the antifibrinolytics and, to a lesser extent, norethisterone which is taken for a minimum of 7 days/cycle. The cost/month at current costs (August, 1989), using the drugs as directed in the British National Formulary is norethisterone £3.30, mefenamic acid £2 and danazol £28. If the prescriptions are for a 3-month period then the drugs bill each year for menorrhagia is about 1 million pounds. Norethisterone and mefenamic acid are cheap, reasonably effective and safe. They are definitely worth a trial in those with dysfunctional uterine bleeding.

The LHRH agonists offer a new approach to the treatment of menorrhagia. They are usually administered either as a nasal spray or as a subcutaneous implant and reduce pituitary LH release with subsequent inhibition of ovulation. Administration of nasal spray reduces the menstrual blood loss although some follicular development may occur with a rise in the cirulating oestradiol[26]. This can lead to breakthrough bleeding which may be heavy and also there is the small risk of the unopposed oestrogen stimulating the endometrium. The subcutaneous implants give more consistent suppression of ovarian oestrogen output[27] and amenorrhoea is the norm after the first month of treatment. Unfortunately post-menopausal side-effects are common and there is a risk of osteoporosis if implants were to be given for more than a few months. Unless an effect on the menstrual blood loss continues to be seen for many months after treatment implants alone are unlikely to have a major role in the treatment of menorrhagia. It may be possible to combine them with agents known to have a bone-sparing effect when they may have a place in women approaching the menopause. However, implants are still a very expensive method of administering agonist and it is unlikely that they will find wider use until the cost is considerably reduced.

HYSTEROSCOPY

The advent of fibre optic telescopes about 20 years ago has increased the applications of hysteroscopy. Recently, it has been used with cryocautery and YAG laser in the treatment of dysfunctional uterine bleeding. Although it may be used on an out-patient basis, less than 1% of gynaecologists are able to use a hysteroscope for either diagnostic or therapeutic purposes.

The results of a recently published pilot study[28] using hysteroscopic transcervical resection of the endometrium are discussed in more detail elsewhere (Chapter 8). This technique, which involves total or partial resection of the endometrium looks promising, although no long-term follow-up or objective measurement of blood loss has yet been published in those with dysfunctional uterine bleeding. De Cherney *et al.* report the use of the cystoscope–resectoscope in patients with intractable uterine bleeding who had blood dyscrasias or were poor anaesthetic risks[29,30]. In those still alive after 5 years most were amenorrhoeic or had light bleeds.

Initially the treatment requires a good anaesthetic and may take up to 2 hours. However, the time decreases with experience and possibly it might be performed under local anaesthesia in selected cases. The length of stay in hospital is short and the women return to work within 2 to 3 weeks. This compares well with hysterectomy where the time off work is frequently 2–3 months. The possible complications of the procedure are uterine perforation, adhesion formation within the uterine cavity, infection and blood loss. Blood loss may be similar to that occurring after hysterectomy but as yet it is too early to give the incidence of complications. Alternatively, endometrial ablation can be performed using hysteroscopic laser ablation[31]. The advantages over endometrial resection have not as yet been evaluated. The equipment required is very expensive and the risk of uterine perforation is probably greater with the potential of damage to bowel or bladder. Loffer advocates a non–touch technique[32] which he finds safer, quicker (30–40 min) and only slightly less effective than the touch technique originally described[32]. However, Davis[33], in a recently published paper, found a combined technique effective in only 52% of patients although Goldrath[34], in a much larger series, reports a 96% success rate. Long-term follow–up is required which utilizes menstrual blood loss for objective assessment.

CONCLUSIONS

The aim of treatment of menorrhagia is to improve the quality of life since it is rarely a life threatening condition. I am not aware of any studies which look at the long-term effects of hysterectomy in this way, probably because there are so many confounding variables. It is much easier to assess the success of other treatments by objectively measuring the menstrual blood loss. However, as I mentioned above, the change in the blood loss does not appear to correlate with patient satisfaction with the treatment. This may be because patients are aware of fluid and not blood loss and also because, with the end of child-bearing, periods are just a nuisance. Even if the gynaecologist has objective evidence that a treatment is working, unless the patient is happy they will refuse to continue with it. Thus our aim must be to continue looking for that safe, effective, acceptable and cheap treatment for dysfunctional uterine bleeding.

REFERENCES

1. Cohen, B.J.B. and Gibor, Y. (1980). Anaemia and Menstrual blood loss. *Obstet. Gynecol. Surv.*, **35**, 597–618
2. Royal College of General Practitioners (1986). Office of Population Censuses and Surveys. Department of Health & Social Security. *Morbidity Statistics from General Practice*. (London: HMSO)
3. Chimbira, T.H., Anderson, A.B.M. and Turnbull, A.C. (1980). Relation between measured menstrual blood loss and patient's subjective assessment of loss, duration of bleeding, number of sanitary towels used, uterine weight and endometrial surface area. *Br. J. Obstet. Gynaecol.*, **87**, 603–9
4. Rybo, G. (1966). Clinical and experimental studies on menstrual blood loss. *Acta Obstet. Gynecol. Scand.*, **45**, suppl. 1–23
5. Fraser, I.S., Pearse, C. and Shearman, R.P. (1981). Efficacy of mefenamic acid in patients with the complaint of menorrhagia. *Obstet. Gynecol.*, **58**, 543–51
6. Cole, S.K., Billewicz, W.Z. and Thomson, A.M. (1971). Sources of variation in menstrual blood loss. *J. Obstet. Gynaecol. Br. Cwlth.*, **78**, 933–9
7. Webb, C. (1983). A study of recovery from hysterectomy. In Wilson-Barnett, J. (ed.) *Nursing Research – Studies in Patient Care*, pp. 7–22 (Bristol: Wiley)
8. Dicker, R.C., Greenspan, J.R. and Strauss, L.T. (1982). Complications of abdominal and vaginal hysterectomy among women of reproductive age in the United States. *Am. J. Obstet. Gynecol.*, **144**, 841–8
9. Wingo, P.A., Huezo, C.M., Rubin, G.L., Ory, H.W. and Peterson, H.B. (1985). The mortality risk associated with hysterectomy. *Am. J. Obstet. Gynecol.*, **152**, 803–8
10. Smith, S.K., Abel, M.H., Kelly, R.W. and Baird, D.T. (1981). Prostaglandin synthesis in the endometrium of women with ovular dysfunctional uterine bleeding. *Br. J. Obstet. Gynaecol.*, **88**, 434–42
11. Oxford Family Planning Association Study, Oxford Regional Health Authority: Hospital Activity Analysis
12. Coulter, A., McPherson, K. and Vessey, M. (1988). Do British women undergo too many or too few hysterectomies? *Soc.Sci.Med.*, **27**,987–94
13. Bunker, J.P. and Brown, B.W. (1974). The physician–patient as an informed consumer of surgical services. *N. Engl. J. Med.*, **290**, 1051–5
14. McPherson, K., Strong, P.M., Epstein, A. and Jones, L. (1981). Regional variations in the use of common surgical procedures: within and between England and Wales, Canada and the United States of America. *Soc. Sci. Med.*, **15A**, 273–88
15. Domenighetti, G., Luraschi, P., Casabianca, A., Gutzwiller, F., Spinelli A.,

Pedrinis, E. and Repetto, F. (1988). Effect of information campaign by the mass media on hysterectomy rates. *Lancet*, **2**, 1470–3

16. Filicori, M., Hall, D.A., Loughlin, J.S., Rivier, J., Vale, W. and Crowley, W.F. (1983). A conservative approach to the management of uterine leiomyoma: pituitary desensitization by a luteinizing hormone – releasing hormone analogue. *Am. J. Obstet. Gynecol.*, **147**, 726–7

17. Healy, D.L., Lawson, S.R., Abbot, M., Baird, D.T. and Fraser, H.M. (1986). Toward removing uterine fibroids without surgery: subcutaneous infusion of a luteinizing hormone-releasing hormone agonist commencing in the luteal phase. *J. Clin. Endocrinol. Metab.*, **63**, 619–25

18. Lumsden, M.A., West. C.P. and Baird, D.T. (1987). Goserelin therapy before surgery for uterine fibroids. *Lancet*, **2**, 36–7

19. Haynes P.J., Anderson, A.B.M. and Turnbull, A.C. (1979). Patterns of menstrual blood loss in menorrhagia. *Res. Clin. Forums*, **1**, 73–8

20. Cameron, I.T., Haining, R., Lumsden, M.A., Thomas, V.R. and Smith, S.K. (1989). The effects of mefenamic acid and norethisterone on measured menstrual blood loss. *Obstet. Gynecol.* (submitted for publication)

21. Dockeray, C.J., Sheppard, B.L. and Bonnar, J. (1989). Comparison between mefenamic acid and danazol in the treatment of established menorrhagia. *Br. J. Obstet. Gynaecol.*, **96**, 840–4

22. Chimbira, T.H., Anderson, A.B., Naish, C., Cope, E. and Turnbull, A.C. (1980). Reduction of menstrual blood loss by danazol in unexplained menorrhagia: lack of effect of placebo. *Br. J. Obstet. Gynaecol.*, **87**, 1152–8

23. Nilsson, L. And Rybo, G. (1971). Treatment of menorrhagia. *Am. J. Obstet. Gynecol.*, **110**, 713–19

24. Rydin, E. and Lundberg, P.O. (1976). Tranexamic acid and intracranial thrombosis. *Lancet*, **2**, 49

25. Harrison, R.F. and Campbell, S. (1976). A double blind trial of ethamsylate in the treatment of primary and intra-uterine device menorrhagia. *Lancet*, **2**, 283–5

26. Shaw, R.W. and Fraser, H.M. (1984). Use of a superactive luteinizing hormone-releasing hormone (LHRH) agonist in the treatment of menorrhaga. *Br. J. Obstet. Gynaecol.*, **91**, 913–16

27. West, C.P. and Baird, D.T. (1986). Suppression of ovarian activity by Zoladex depot (ICI 118630), a long acting luteinising hormone releasing hormone agonist analogue. *Clin. Endocrinol.*, **26**, 213–20

28. Magos, A.L., Baumann, R. and Turnbull, A.C. (1989). Transcervical resection of endometrium in women with menorrhagia. *Br. Med. J.*, **298**, 1209–12

29. De Cherney, A.H. and Polan, M.L. (1983). Hysteroscopic management of intra-uterine lesions and intractable uterine bleeding. *Obstet. Gynecol.*, **61**, 392–7

30. De Cherney, A.H., Diamond, M.P., Lavy, G. and Polan, M.L. (1987). Endometrial ablation for intractable uterine bleeding – hysteroscopic resection. *Obstet. Gynecol.*, **70**, 668–70

31. Goldrath, M.H., Fuller, T.A. and Segal, S. (1981). Laser photovaporisation of endometrium for treatment of menorrhagia. *Am. J. Obstet. Gynecol.*, **140**, 14–19

32. Loffer, F.D. (1987). Hysteroscopic endometrial ablation with the Nd–Yag laser using a nontouch technique. *Obstet. Gynecol.*, **69**, 679–82

33. Davis, J.A. (1989). Hysteroscopic endometrial ablation with the neodymium–YAG laser. *Br. J. Obstet. Gynaecol.*, **96**, 928–32

34. Goldrath, M.H. (1986). Hysteroscopic laser ablation of the endometrium. In Sharp, F. and Jordan, J.A., (eds). *Gynaecological Laser Surgery*, pp. 253–265. Proceedings of the 15th Study Group of the RCOG, London, 1985. (New York: Perinatology Press)

8

Endometrial ablation techniques

A.L. Magos

Attempts at endometrial destruction with the aim of producing a therapeutic type of Asherman's syndrome in cases of abnormal menstruation have been made by a variety of techniques[1]. Early trials involved the intrauterine application of cytotoxic chemicals (e.g. quinacrine, methyl cyanoacrylate, oxalic acid, paraformaldehyde, 100% ethanol, 10% formalin)[2-4], intracavity radium[5,6], superheated steam[7], autologous fibroblasts[8-10], and cryosurgery (eg. freon, nitrous oxide)[11-15] but were generally unsucessful and have been abandoned. All the above techniques were carried out blindly with the tendency for incomplete treatment which, together with the remarkable powers of endometrial regeneration if the basal layer is left intact[16], meant that the therapeutic results were inconsistent.

More recently, hysteroscopic techniques of laser ablation and endometrial diathermy or resection have been described. These methods hold out more promise partly because they are carried out under direct vision making skip lesions less likely. As with the earlier methods, endometrial destruction is only suitable for women who have completed their families, and in whom the endometrium is histologically normal and the uterine cavity is not grossly enlarged. Pretreatment with high doses of danazol for 3–4 weeks prevents endometrial growth and makes the operation by either method technically considerably easier.

LASER ABLATION

In 1981 Goldrath *et al.* reported the first series of 22 hysteroscopic laser ablations[17], and considerable support is now available concerning the efficacy of this approach[18-26]. Of the currently available sources of laser energy the neodymium:yttrium–aluminium–garnet (Nd:YAG) laser is optimal for intrauterine surgery as it can be delivered along a flexible fibre (an advantage with the awkward shape of the endometrial cavity), can be transmitted through liquid media (as used for uterine distension in operative hysteroscopy), and the depth of tissue penetration can be controlled (a relative protection against uterine perforation). Either rigid or flexible telescopes can be used to apply the laser energy to the endometrium.

The target effect includes the sequence of warming, coagulation, evaporation and carbonization, tissue destruction typically occurring to a depth of 4–5 mm. Although the mean endometrial thickness after short-term danazol treatment is only 1.2 mm, glandular elements are almost invariably present deeper in the myometrium and ablation (or resection) should therefore include 2.5–3 mm of myometrium[27]. At the power settings used for endometrial ablation heat transmission through the myometrium is not clinically important, additional protection being afforded by the continuous flow of cool irrigation fluid as well as circulating blood flow[17,28].

Three techniques have been described: touch technique, non-touch technique, and a combination of the two. In the touch technique the tip of the quartz fibre, which may be capped with a sapphire tip, is dragged across the endometrium with resultant vaporization and the production of deep furrows down to myometrium. In the non-touch technique the endometrium is merely coagulated, an effect that is characterized by blanching and swelling. The non-touch technique appears safer with regards to peroperative fluid overload or postoperative bleeding but is not as effective in improving menstrual flow as the touch technique. In a recent series, the duration for ablation using the touch technique ranged from 45 to 120 min, with a mean procedure time of 81.7 minutes[26]. Tubal ligation is no longer thought to be required as the uterine cavity undergoes fibrosis and contracts following ablation with blockage of the utero-tubal junction within 6 months[18].

The results of laser endometrial ablation in over 350 women in the USA over a follow-up of up to 6 years have been well reviewed by

Table 1 Results of Nd:YAG laser endometrial ablation (adapted from Loffer[25])

	Goldrath[18]	*Loffer*[22]	*Multicentre study*
Number of cases	216	60	45
Operative complications (%)	>4	0	7
Maximum follow-up (years)	6	4.5	1
Results not known	44	5	22
Amenorrhoea (%)	48	20	4
Hypomenorrhoea (%)	48	49	74
Normal flow (%)	12	20	13
Failed (%)	2	11	9
Hysterectomy (%)	3	5	4

Loffer[25]. Apart from the differential effects of touch and non-touch techniques already noted, he concluded that menstrual flow is improved in 89–98% with only 3–8% of women coming to hysterectomy (Table 1). Similarly encouraging results have been reported from France with an ultimate hysterectomy rate of 10%[24].

A recent detailed study in the UK, admittedly of only 25 women, has cast some doubts on the efficacy of laser endometrial ablation with amenorrhoea in only three (12%) cases despite use of the touch technique, with 12 (48%) women coming to hysterectomy[26]. Learning curve aside, considerably better results were obtained in the latter half of the study when a high power setting was used (80 W), and this observation may be the key to success. It has also been shown that poorer results are associated with younger age, submucous fibroids, uterine cavity >10 cm in length, and perhaps adenomyosis[25]. It is of interest that histological examination of hysterectomy specimens some time after ablation typically shows myometrium covered with a single layer of cuboidal epithelium showing minimal inflammation or carbonization[18].

ENDOMETRIAL DIATHERMY/RESECTION

Intrauterine surgery with a resectoscope for the treatment of focal lesions such as fibroids, septa and even benign mesodermal tumours has been reported over the past 10 years[29-34]. More extensive surgery to the entire endometrial surface was first described in 1983, when DeCherney treated 11 women with intractable uterine bleeding resistant to other therapies with emergency endometrial diathermy[35]. Four years later the series was extended to 21 cases, all but three of the patients suffering from blood dyscrasias or other serious illnesses[36]. Excluding three women who died within 6 months of surgery from their primary disease, most survivors were either amenorrhoeic or had slight spotting during the follow-up of up to 5 years, with one patient requiring a second ablation.

Endometrial diathermy thus seems an effective surgical solution to uncontrollable uterine haemorrhage, but the above results may not necessarily apply to healthy women with menorrhagia. The studies were retrospective, uterine bleeding was not recorded in any way before or after surgery, and most importantly, concurrent drug therapy for conditions such as leukaemia and aplastic anaemia which may themselves affect ovarian function, were not accounted for. The first prospective study of transcervical resection of the endometrium (TCRE) in otherwise healthy women with menorrhagia was published in 1989[37].

Our technique of TCRE is conceptually similar to transurethral resection of the prostate in men and is currently performed with a 26 French gauge unmodified continuous flow resectoscope fitted with a 4 mm forward-oblique telescope. The resectoscope is introduced into the uterus after dilating the cervix to 10 mm. The use of electrocautery means that the uterus must be distended with a non-electrolyte solution, and we use sterile 1.5% glycine infused at a pressure of 100 mmHg (Dextran 70 is an alternative); uterine irrigation is achieved by continuous suction of the glycine solution via the outer sheath of the resectoscope at a pressure of 50–100 mmHg, the balance between in-and out-flow being carefully monitored during surgery.

We attach a small video camera to the eye-piece and operate off the video monitor which has the advantages of increasing operator comfort, magnifying the operative field, and is of course excellent for teaching purposes. After careful inspection of the cavity and myomectomy in cases with submucous fibroids, the endometrium is systematically excised down to the superficial layer of myometrium using a mixed diathermy current of 100 W for cutting and 50 W for coagulation. Our usual operative sequence starts at the cornua and fundus, followed by the posterior uterine wall, lateral walls and finally the anterior wall.

Table 2 Intrauterine surgery in Oxford (1.8.88–31.7.89)

Total TCRE ± myomectomy	40
Partial TCRE ± myomectomy	10
Myomectomy only	9
Failed	1
Total	60

Depending on the patient's wishes for amenorrhoea or hypomenorrhoea, the endometrium is resected either over the entire cavity (total resection) or to within 1 cm of the isthmus (partial resection) respectively. Care is taken not to resect too deep as this can result in the opening of relatively large vessels and intraoperative haemorrhage. Laparoscopy is not carried out routinely unless tubal ligation is intended; as with laser ablation, we do not feel that sterilization is essential.

In the 12 months from 1st August 1988 to 31st July 1989 we performed a total of 60 intrauterine surgical procedures, including 50 TCREs on 48 patients with menorrhagia, two women undergoing repeat resections (Table 2). The mean age of the study group was 41.7 years (range 25–54). Fibroids were not a contraindication to resection unless uterine size exceeded the equivalent of a 12 weeks pregnancy. All women accepted that the treatment would make them sterile. We now routinely suppress endometrial proliferation with danazol 200 mg tds for at least 3 weeks preoperatively.

The mean operative time for the first 50 cases was 43.5 min (range 15–100), and depended greatly on the size of the uterine cavity, thickness of the endometrium and presence of fibroids (Figure 1). The total amount of glycine solution infused into the uterus was very variable, the mean volume in these 50 procedures being 5.15 l (range 1.5–20.9), with a mean deficit at the end of surgery of 0.54 l (range 0.1–4.35). Only one woman developed clinical signs of fluid overload in the immediate postoperative period which responded promptly to diuretics; generally, fluid absorption was least when the procedure was short and the Fallopian tubes had previously been ligated (Figure 2). Other complications were equally unusual, the most serious being two women who sustained a uterine perforation during surgery early in our series; one had an acutely retroflexed uterus which made insertion of the rigid hysteroscope difficult, the other an incompetent cervix which prevented adequate

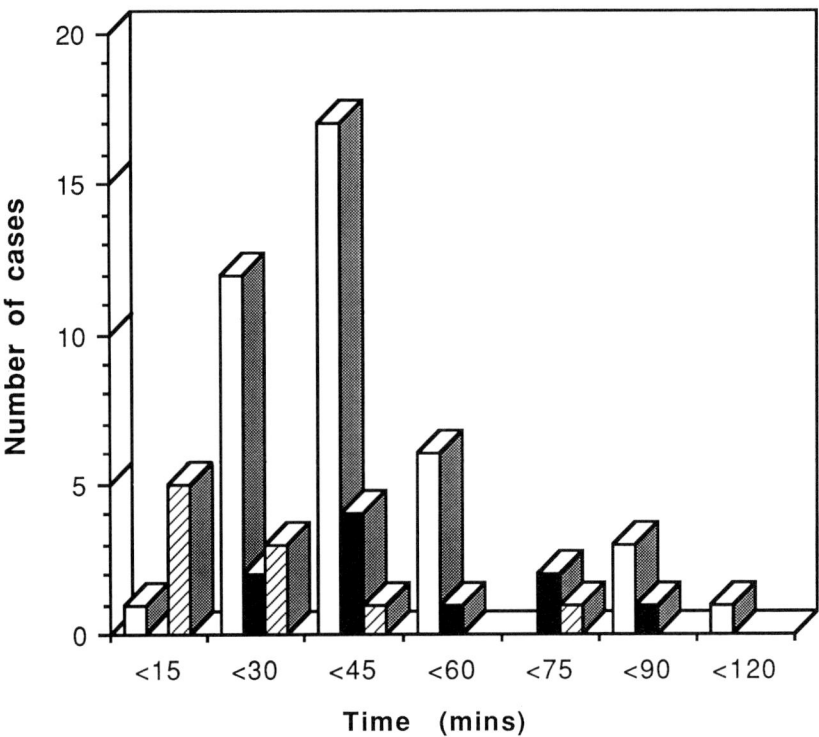

Figure 1 Operative time for intrauterine surgery; comparison between total TCRE (open blocks), partial TCRE (filled blocks) and myomectomy (hatched blocks)

uterine distension (Table 3). As safety precautions, we now ensure that the tubal ostia are identified before proceeding with resection and would insert a cerclage into the cervix if fluid leak from the cervix was excessive.

Recovery from TCRE is fast, and indeed patients are now routinely discharged from hospital on the day of surgery. Everyday activities and work are generally resumed within 3 weeks, but there are some who are back to normal after only a few days (Table 4). Hysteroscopy 3 months after resection typically shows fibrosis of the uterine cavity which is sometimes completely obliterated. Interestingly, even in women who are amenorrhoeic, microscopic deposits of endometrium can often be found in biopsies taken from the new cavity.

As for the menstrual effects, amenorrhoea is achieved in 40–50% of patients after total resection, there being no tendency for a recurrence of

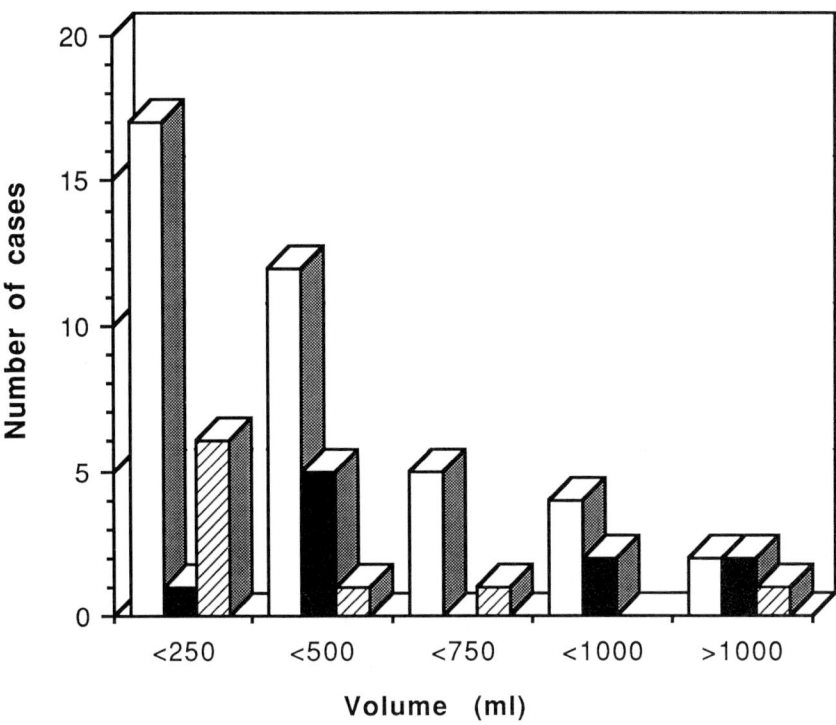

Figure 2 Absorption of glycine irrigant during intrauterine surgery; comparison between total TCRE (open blocks), partial TCRE (filled blocks) and myomectomy (hatched blocks)

Table 3 Complications of TCRE (*n*=51)

Uterine perforation	2
Postoperative pyrexia	2
Urinary retention	1
Urinary tract infection	1
Intrauterine infection	1
Fluid over-load	1

Table 4 Recovery after TCRE (expressed as mean and range)

Hospital stay (days)	1.2 (0.0–13)
Normal activities (weeks)	1.7 (0.5–4)
Work (weeks)	2.6 (0.5–6)

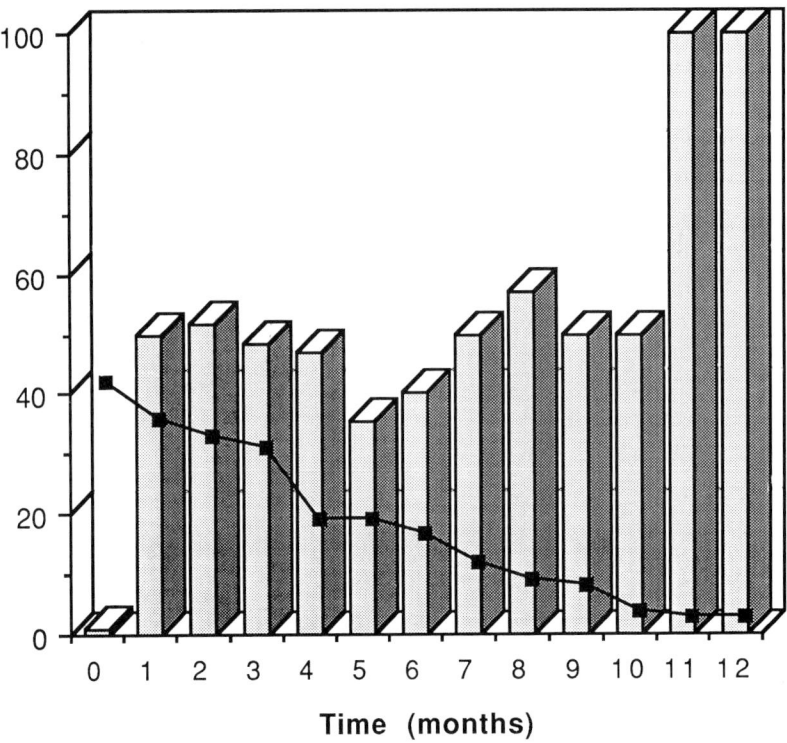

Figure 3 Amenorrhoea after total transcervical resection of the endometrium; ■, number of cases, bars indicate % amenorrhoeic

menstruation with time (Figure 3). Those who continue to bleed after total resection generally develop relative hypomenorrhoea with a reduction in not only the duration of bleeding and amount of blood loss, but also the amount of pain experienced during menstruation (Figure 4). The benefits of partial TCRE are equally consistent but not as great (Figure 5). These subjective impressions have been confirmed by the objective measure of menstrual blood loss using the alkaline haematin method; data on the first 17 patients monitored shows an average improvement in blood loss of over 91% (Table 5). Overall, the great majority of our patients were very satisfied with the results of resection and only three (6%) have requested hysterectomy subsequently (Table 6).

INTRAUTERINE SURGERY UNDER INTRAVENOUS SEDATION

Sedation techniques are already widely employed for diagnostic and therapeutic gastrointestinal and bronchial endoscopy. The autonomic nerve supply of the uterus and resultant relative insensitivity to touching, cutting or burning, means that intrauterine surgery without general anaesthesia should be equally possible. Minor hysteroscopic procedures using relatively narrow instruments have already been described under these conditions[21,30], but we have found that extensive intrauterine surgery can also be carried out[38]. We have performed 19 endometrial resections under intravenous sedation (Table 7), and indeed we now routinely perform TCREs as an out-patient procedure in the endoscopy suite.

Table 5 Menstrual blood loss measurements after TCRE ($n = 17$)

	Mean	*Minimum*	*Maximum*
Before (ml)	201.9	13.0	528.5
After (ml)	17.2	0.0	58.3
% Improvement	+91.5	−15.4	+100.0

Table 6 Results of TCRE ($n=49$)

Failed	1 (2%)
Satisfied	43 (88%)
Repeat resection	2 (4%)
Hysterectomy	3 (6%)

Table 7 Anaesthesia for intrauterine surgery ($n = 60$); GA, general anaesthesia or LA, local anaesthesia

	GA	LA + sedation
Total TCRE	29	12 (29.3%)
Partial TCRE	8	2 (20.0%)
Myomectomy	2	7 (77.8%)
All cases	39	21 (35.0%)

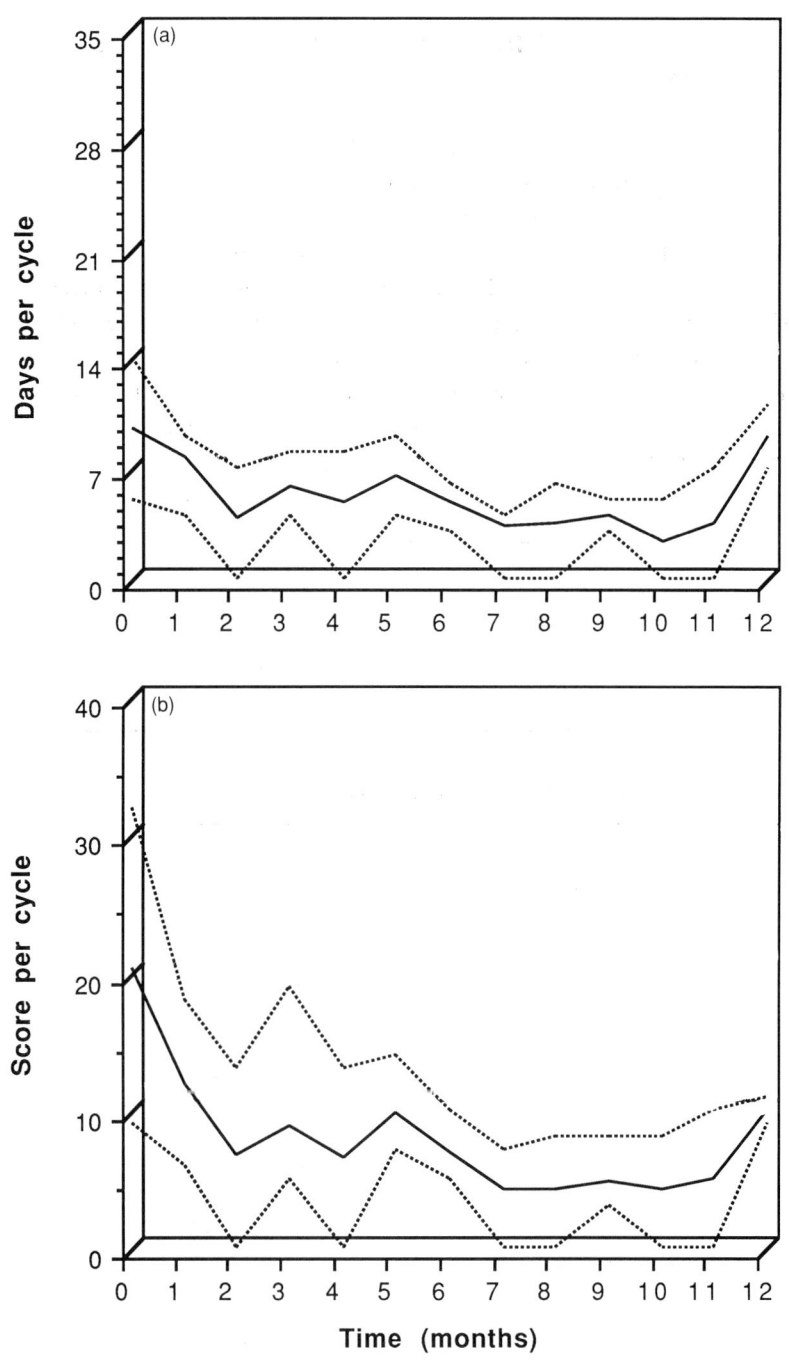

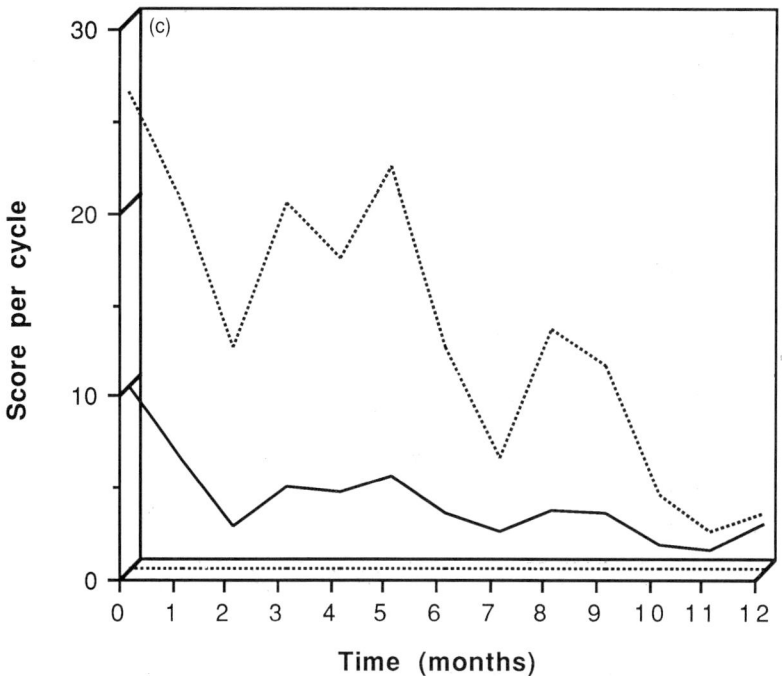

Figure 4 Effect of total transcervical resection of the endometrium (a) on the duration of menstruation; (b) on menstrual scores [blood loss scored daily on a scale of 0 to 3 (none to heavy)]; and (c) on menstrual pain scores [pain scored daily on a scale of 0 to 3 (none to severe)]. Solid lines indicate mean values, upper dotted lines the maxima and lower dotted lines the minima

Our current protocol involves admitting the patient in time for premedication with temazepam 20 mg and mefenamic acid 500 mg 1 h before surgery. In the endoscopy suite, light sedation is achieved with small doses of intravenous midazolam, and analgesia with a combination of para- and intracervical lignocaine with adrenaline and intravenous fentanyl. Heart rate, electrocardiogram and arterial oxygen saturation are monitored continuously during surgery, facial oxygen being given if there is evidence of hypoventilation. Patients remain fully co-operative during surgery, some even choosing to watch their operation 'live' on the video monitor, and are discharged home 3–4 h afterwards when fully conscious and orientated. Most women so far treated have been pleased about the avoidance of not only hysterectomy but also general anaesthesia.

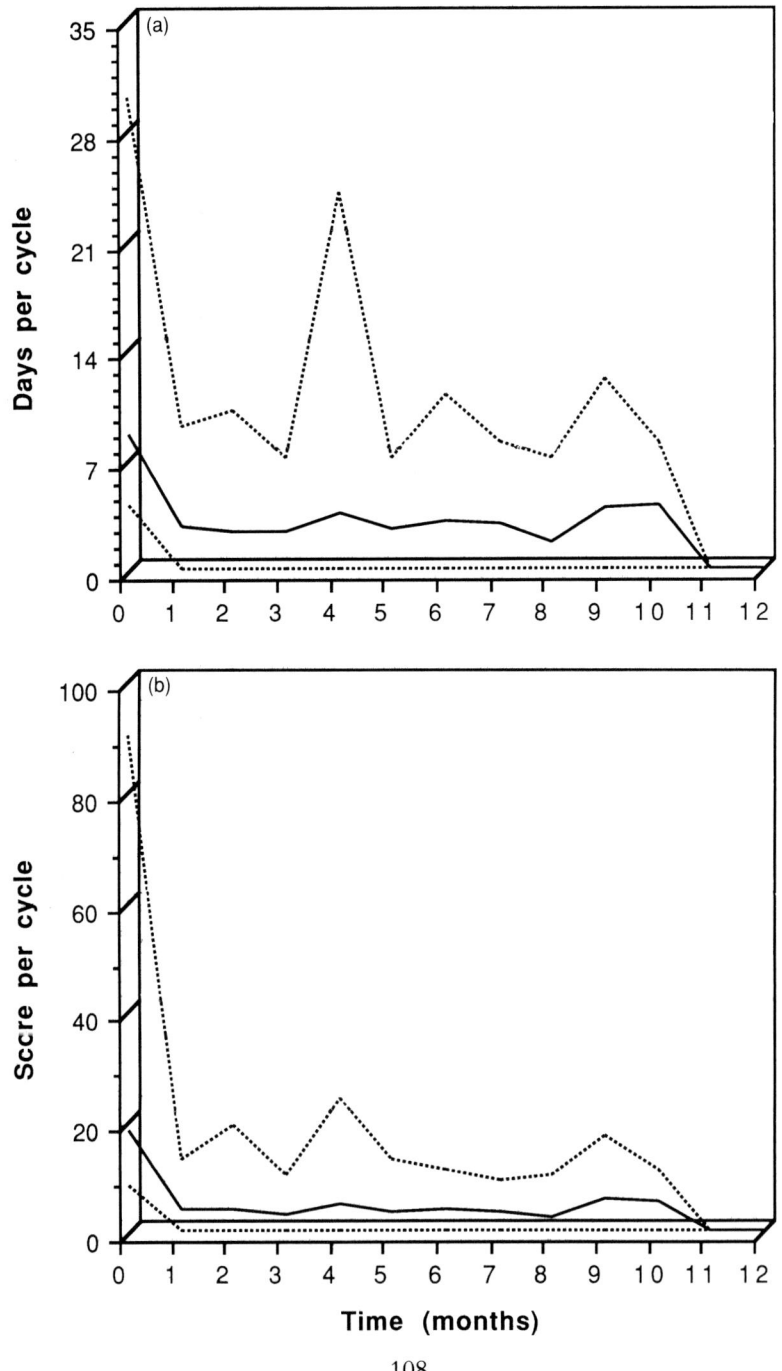

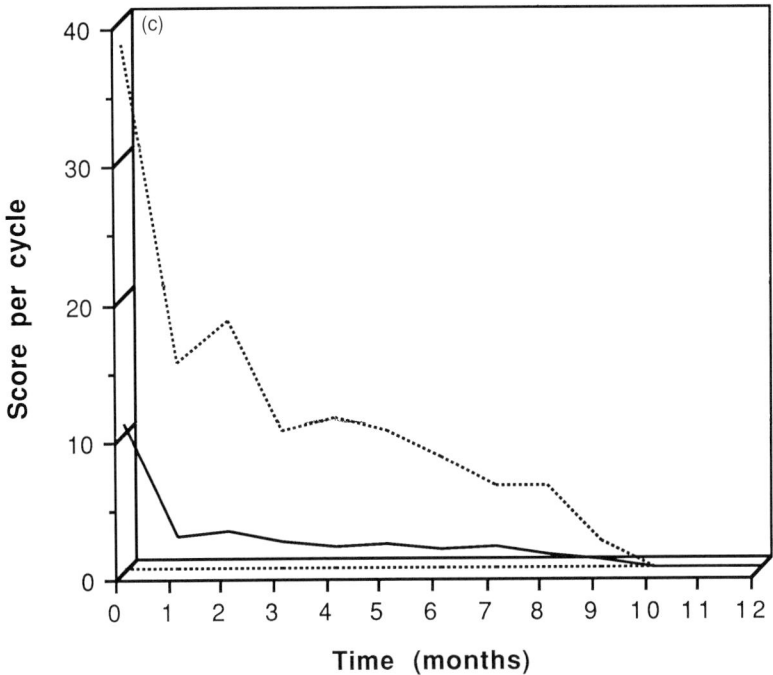

Figure 5 Effect of partial transcervical resection of the endometrium (a) on the duration of menstruation; (b) on menstrual scores [blood loss scored daily on a scale of 0 to 3 (none to heavy)]; and (c) on menstrual pain scores [pain scored daily on a scale of 0 to 3 (none to severe)]. Solid lines indicate mean values, upper dotted lines the maxima and lower dotted lines the minima

RISKS OF INTRAUTERINE SURGERY

Endometrial destruction by either of the techniques described is not for the novice, but should be an extension of basic skills learnt for diagnostic procedures. The obvious risks of extensive intrauterine surgery include haemorrhage, infection and in particular uterine perforation. The use of large volumes of irrigating fluid is associated with the dangers of excessive absorption resulting in fluid overload, hypertension, hyponatraemia, neurological symptoms, haemolysis and even death, collectively known as the TUR (transurethral resection) syndrome. All these complications however seem to be relatively uncommon[18].

109

There have only been two reports looking formally at fluid dynamics during endometrial surgery. Morrison *et al.* investigated 12 women undergoing laser ablation using 0.9% saline as the uterine irrigant[39]. In their study the mean volume of uterine irrigant absorbed was 2.5 l (maximum 10.5), fluid absorption being accompanied by a significant rise in central venous pressure and serum chloride and significant decrease in plasma total protein, albumin and haematocrit.

We looked at the absorption of glycine irrigating solution during TCRE in 10 women[40] and found that fluid absorption was considerably less with this procedure, with a mean volume of only 0.64 l (range 0.1–2.03). There was an inverse linear correlation between the volume of irrigant absorbed and fall in plasma sodium ($r=-0.77$, $p < 0.02$), intraoperative hyponatraemia affecting two of the three women with fluid deficits in excess of 0.9 l. As with the previous study, changes in plasma sodium were paralleled by falls in the serum concentration of total protein, albumin, haemoglobin and packed cell volume. There was also evidence of delayed intravascular haemolysis but all parameters returned to normal spontaneously within 24 h. In contrast to Morrison *et al.*[39], our results suggested that transtubal loss and consequent peritoneal absorption is an important route of fluid loss during TCRE. Both studies emphasize the importance of careful monitoring of fluid balance during hysteroscopic surgery.

ABLATE OR RESECT?

Accepting that TCRE is a more recent procedure with a shorter follow-up, the results so far suggest that laser ablation and endometrial resection are of comparable efficacy in producing amenorrhoea and hypomenorrhoea. Both techniques have advantages and disadvantages (Table 8), but in the cost conscious climate of the present health care system, the lesser capital outlay and faster operating time associated with TCRE must weigh heavily in its favour as the preferred surgical option.

HYSTEROSCOPIC SURGERY OR HYSTERECTOMY?

Endometrial destruction by laser or electrocautery seems an attractive alternative to both long-term drug therapy and hysterectomy for the

Table 8 Comparison of laser and resectoscope surgery

	Laser	*Resectoscope*
Precision	+++	++
Safety	++	+
Speed	+	++
Cost	+	+++
Histology	+	+++
Efficacy	???	???

Worst + <————> +++ best

management of the common complaint of abnormal menstruation. Hysteroscopic treatment is associated with a much shorter hospital stay, faster recovery, definite financial savings, and menstruation is almost universally improved to a clinically meaningful degree. On the debit side, amenorrhoea cannot be guaranteed with present techniques and long-term morbidity is as yet unknown. Of concern are the recent findings of a large retrospective comparison of transurethral resection of the prostate with open prostatectomy in men showing a small but significantly increased risk of dying from cardiovascular causes for up to 8 years after the endoscopic procedure[41]. While the results of this study cannot be applied directly to hysteroscopic endometrial surgery, it is important to provide patients with all the facts (Table 9). Ultimately, a formal comparison with traditional treatments must be the judge of the therapeutic role of endometrial destruction.

CONCLUSIONS

There seems little doubt that hysteroscopic intrauterine surgery, particularly destruction or excision of the endometrium, is set to dramatically change everyday gynaecological practice. However, the indications and contraindication, limitations and above all operative risks of the techniques must be appreciated. Hysteroscopy is technically quite different from laparoscopy, and expertise with the latter is no guarantee of success with the former. Training in hysteroscopic surgery is an essential prerequisite to ensure the safety and proper care of our patients. It is a technique well worth learning.

Table 9 Comparison between hysterectomy and hysteroscopic endometrial destruction

	Advantages	*Disadvantages*
Total hysterectomy	Amenorrhoea certain Suitable for any size of uterus Abdominal contents can be inspected Other surgery possible (e.g. oophorectomy) No risk of uterine or cervical malignancy Treats unsuspected uterine malignancy	Major surgery Requires general anaesthestic Abdominal scar Hospital stay 5–7 days Convalescence 6–8 weeks ?Depression ?Earlier menopause ?Psychosexual problems ?Functional bowel disorders ?Ischaemic heart disease
Endometrial surgery	Minor surgery Suitable for women unfit for general anaesthesia No scars Short hospital stay Quick convalescence Possibility for repeat procedure ?Uterus retained	Menstruation in 50% Not suitable for grossly enlarged uterus Abdominal contents cannot be inspected Other surgery not possible Risk of uterine or cervical malignancy Does not treat unsuspected uterine malignancy ?Unknown complications

ACKNOWLEDGEMENTS

The author is grateful to the ODHIF Trust Deed, Sir Samual Scott of Yews Trust, and Oxford Hospital Services Development Trust for grants towards the cost of our equipment and investigations; Rimmer Brothers of London for loan of the remaining instruments; and my colleagues Ralf Baumann, Margaret Rees and Professor Sir Alexander Turnbull for their invaluable help and support.

REFERENCES

1. Asherman, J.G. (1948). Amenorrhoea traumatica (atretica). *J. Obstet. Gynaecol. Br. Emp.*, **55**, 23–30
2. Zipper, J.A., Stachetti, E. and Medel, M. (1970). Human fertility control by transvaginal application of quinacrine on the fallopian tube. *Fertil. Steril.*, **21**, 581–9
3. Stevenson, T.C. and Taylor, D.S. (1972). the effect of methyl cyanoacrylate tissue adhesive on the human fallopian tube and endometrium. *J. Obstet. Gynaecol. Br. Cwlth.*, **79**, 1028–39
4. Zipper, J., Medel, M., Pastene, L. and Rivera, M. (1969). Intrauterine instillation of chemical cytotoxic agents for tubal sterilization and treatment of functional metrorrhagias. *Int. J. Fertil.*, **14**, 280–8
5. Rongy, A.J. (1947). Radium therapy in benign uterine bleeding. *J. Mt. Sinai Hosp.*, **14**, 569–75
6. Falconer, B. (1947). The treatment of metropathia haemorrhagica: suggestions for a therapeutic programme. *Acta Obstet. Gynaecol. Scand.*, **27**, 288–96
7. Crossen, R.J. and Crossen, H.S. (1947). Radiation therapy for uterine myoma. *J. Am. Med. Assoc.*, **133**, 593–9
8. Polishnuk, W.Z. and Schenker, J.G. (1973). Induction of intrauterine adhesions in the rabbit with autogenous fibroblast implants. *Am. J. Obstet. Gynecol.*, **115**, 789–94
9. Schenker, J.G., Nicosia, S.V., Polishuk, W.Z. and Garcia, C.R. (1975). An *in-vitro* fibroplast-enriched sponge preparation for induction of intrauterine adhesions. *Israel J. Med. Sci.*, **11**, 849–51
10. Polishuk, W.Z. (1975). Endometrial regeneration and adhesion formation. *S. A. Med. J.*, **49**, 440–2
11. Droegemueller, W., Greer, B. and Makowski, E. (1970). Preliminary observations of cryocoagulation of the endometrium. *Am. J. Obstet. Gynecol.*, **107**, 958–61
12. Droegemueller, W., Greer, B. and Makowski, E. (1971). Cryosurgery in patients with dysfunctional uterine bleeding. *Obstet. Gynecol.*, **38**, 256–8
13. Droegemueller, W., Makowski, E. and Macsalka, R. (1971). Destruction of the endometrium by cryosurgery. *Am. J. Obstet. Gynecol.*, **110**, 467–9
14. Schenker, J. G. and Polishuk, W.Z. (1972). Regeneration of the rabbit endometrium after cryosurgery. *Obstet. Gynecol.*, **40**, 638–45
15. Droegemueller, W., Greer, B.E., Davis, J.R., Makowski, E.L., Chvapil, N. and Pollard, A. (1978). Cryocoagulation of the endometrium at the uterine cornua. *Am. J. Obstet. Gynecol.*, **131**, 1–9
16. Baggish, M.S., Pauerstein, C.J. and Woodruff, J.D. (1967). Role of stroma in

regeneration of endometrial epithelium. *Am. J. Obstet. Gynecol.*, **99**, 459–65

17. Goldrath, M.H., Fuller, T.A. and Segal, S. (1981). Laser photovaporization of endometrium for the treatment of menorrhagia. *Am. J. Obstet. Gynecol.*, **140**, 14–19

18. Goldrath, M.H. (1986). Hysteroscopic laser ablation of the endometrium. In Sharp, F. and Jordan, J.A. (eds). *Gynaecological Laser Surgery:* Proceedings of the Fifteenth Study Group of the Royal College of Obstetricians and Gynaecologists, London, pp. 253–69. (New York: Perinatology Press)

19. Lomano, J.M. (1986). Photocoagulation of the endometrium with the Nd:YAG laser for the treatment of menorrhagia. *J. Reprod. Med.*, **31**, 148–50

20. Daniell, J., Tosh, R. and Meisels, S. (1986). Photodynamic ablation of the endometrium with the Nd:YAG laser hysteroscopically as a treatment for menorrhagia. *Colp. Gynecol. Laser Surg.*, **2**, 43–6

21. Cornier, E. (1986). Traitement hysterofibroscopique ambulatoire des metrorragies rebelles par laser Nd:YAG. J. *Gynecol. Obstet. Biol. Reprod.* (Paris), **15**, 661–4

22. Loffer, F.D. (1987). Hysteroscopic endometrial ablation with the Nd:YAG laser using a non-touch technique. *Obstet. Gynecol.*, **69**, 679–82

23. Baggish, M.S. and Baltoyannis, P. (1988). New techniques for laser ablation of the endometrium in high-risk patients. *Am. J. Obstet. Gynecol.*, **159**, 287–92

24. Cornier, E. (1988). Experience with laser Nd:YAG during hysteroscopy: long term results in the treatment of menorrhagia in 144 cases. Presented at the *IIIrd European Congress on Hysteroscopy and Endoscopic Surgery*, September, Amsterdam

25. Loffer, F.D. (1988). Laser ablation of the endometrium *Obstet. Clin. N. Am.*, **15**, 77–89

26. Davis, J. A. (1989). Hysteroscopic endometrial ablation with the neodymium-YAG laser. *Br. J. Obstet. Gynaecol.*, **96**, 928–32

27. Reid, P.C. and Sharp, F. (1988). Hysteroscopic Nd:YAG endometrial ablation: an *in vitro* and *in vivo* laser-tissue interaction study. Presented at the *IIIrd European Congress on Hysteroscopy and Endoscopic Surgery*, September, Amsterdam

28. Mosely, H., Morris, J.D., McLeod, P.W., Davison, M., Hawthorn, R.J.S. and Davis, J.A. (1987). Thermal effects of intra-uterine Nd YAG laser endometrial ablation. *Lasers Med. Sci.*, **2**, 77–89

29. Neuwirth, R.S. (1978). A new technique for and additional experience with hysteroscopic resection of submucous fibroids. *Am. J. Obstet. Gynecol.*, **131**, 91–4

30. Hallez, J.-P., Netter, A. and Cartier, R. (1987). Methodical intrauterine

resection. *Am. J. Obstet. Gynecol.*, **156**, 1080–4

31. Chervenak, F.A. and Neuwirth, R.S. (1981). Hysteroscopic resection of the uterine septum. *Am. J. Obstet. Gynecol.*, **141**, 351–3

32. DeCherny, A.H., Russell, J.B., Graebe, R.A. and Polan, M.L. (1986). Resectoscopic management of mullerian fusion defects. *Fertil. Steril.*, **45**, 726–8

33. Rock, J.A., Murphy, A.A. and Cooper, W.H. (1987). Resectoscopic techniques for the lysis of a class V: complete uterine septum. *Fertil. Steril.*, **48**, 495–6

34. Haning, R.V., Harkins, P.G. and Uehling, D.T. (1980). Preservation of fertility by transcervical resection of a benign mesodermal uterine tumor with a resectoscope and glycine distending medium. *Fertil. Steril.*, **33**, 209–10

35. DeCherney, A. and Polan, M.L. (1983). Hysteroscopic management of intrauterine lesions and intractable uterine bleeding. *Obstet. Gynecol.*, **61**, 392–7

36. DeCherney, A.H., Diamond, M.P., Lavy, G. and Polan, M.L. (1987). Endometrial ablation for intractable uterine bleeding: hysteroscopic resection. *Obstet. Gynecol.*, **70**, 668–70

37. Magos, A.L., Baumann, R. and Turnbull, A.C. (1989). Transcervical resection of the endometrium in women with menorrhagia. *Br. Med. J.*, **298**, 1209–12

38. Magos, A.L., Baumann, R., Cheung, K. and Turnbull, A.C. (1989). Intrauterine surgery under intravenous sedation; as an out-patient alternative to hysterectomy. *Lancet*, **2**, 925–6

39. Morrison, L.M.M., Davis, J. and Sumner, D. (1989). Absorption of irrigating fluid during laser photocoagulation of the endometrium in the treatment of menorrhagia. *Br.J. Obstet. Gynaecol.*, **96**, 346–52

40. Baumann, R., Magos, A.L., Kay, J.D.S. and Turnbull, A.C. (1989). Absorption of glycine irrigating solution during transcervical resection of the endometrium. *Br. Med. J.*, **300**, 304–5

41. Roos, N.P., Wennberg, J.E., Malenka, D.J., Fisher, E.S., McPherson, K., Andersen, T.F., Cohen, M.M. and Ramsey, E. (1989). Mortality and reoperation after opan and transurethral resection of the prostate for benign prostatic hyperplasia. *N. Engl. J. Med.*, **320**, 1120–4

DISCUSSION

Prof. S.K. Smith   Partial and total resection were mentioned. Which is the correct one to do?

Mr A.L. Magos   It is up to the patient. We ask the patient what she wants, whether she wants to have no periods ideally or light periods. If she says no periods, which the majority of our patients do say, then we do a complete resection trying to resect the entire endometrial cavity. If she wants light periods we make sure we leave a little bit of endometrium behind.

Miss G.C.L. Lachelin   Is there any worry about trapping tissue and then someone getting a carcinoma developing which would not present?

Mr A.L. Magos   That question in one of the worries, which is why I think a long-term study is very important and perhaps a long-term comparison with hysterectomy. However, we are removing the majority of the endometrium and that should reduce the risk of endometrial cancer.

Mr S.M. Wood   Complications were mentioned but I was surprised that there was no mention of intra- or post-operative bleeding.

Mr A.L. Magos   There can be bleeding, or excessive bleeding, if the resection goes too deep because there are some big blood vessels deep in the myometrium. This is why one should go to only 2 or 3 mm depth. If it should happen, the resectoscope is a very good instrument for stopping bleeding, one can just press on the blood vessel, apply coagulation current, and the bleeding will stop.

Mr T.M. Coltart   Would Mr Magos feel confident giving unopposed oestrogen hormone replacement therapy to stop osteoporosis?

Mr A.L. Magos   I would not at the moment. One of the things we do with our patients routinely is to hysteroscope them 3 months after resection. The interesting finding there, apart from the very small uterine cavity, is that even those who do not bleed, who are amenorrhoeic, if we do a biopsy 50% at least will have endometrial glands in the biopsy.

9

The use of prostaglandin synthetase inhibitors in dysfunctional uterine bleeding

C.J. Dockeray

Prostaglandin synthetase inhibitors (PGSIs) are non-steroidal, anti-inflammatory analgesics which can be divided into two main groupings: the aryl carboxylic acids, including the salicylic acids (aspirin) and fenamates (flufenamic acid, mefenamic acid, sodium meclofenamate); and the aryl alkanoic acids, including the aryl propionic acids (ibuprofen, ketoprofen and naproxen); the indole acetic acids (indomethacin) and phenylacetic acid (diclofenac sodium).

PGSIs, including mefenamic acid, naproxen, ibuprofen and diclofenac sodium, have been shown to be effective in reducing excessive menstrual bleeding in women with intrauterine devices[1-5]. However, studies relating to the effect of PGSIs on women with dysfunctional uterine bleeding are almost entirely confined to the effect of the fenamate mefenamic acid[6-10]; the beneficial effects having been first reported by Anderson and her colleagues in 1976.

The precise mode of action of PGSIs in reducing menstrual blood loss is not fully understood. They inhibit the synthesis of cyclic endoperoxides in the microsomal fraction of the cell through their inhibitory action on the enzyme cyclo-oxygenase. Different PGSIs, however, give different responses not only in degree of enzyme inhibition but also in respect to different organs[11]. Within the uterus ibuprofen inhibits $PGF_{2\alpha}$ to a greater extent then PGE_2, whereas both are suppressed equally by naproxen[12]. The fenamates sodium meclofenamate

117

and mefenamic acid have recently been shown to inhibit the binding of PGE_2 to its specific receptor in the myometrium[13]. Whether this dual effect of the fenamates on prostaglandin synthesis and binding applies to other PGSIs has yet to be determined.

As advances in therapy slowly evolve through clinic research, our prescribing habits are ultimately influenced by the medical and pharmaceutical literature purporting the advantages of a particular product. When evaluating studies for the treatment of menorrhagia it is appropriate to consider the following.

STUDY DESIGN

Studies based on subjective assessment of blood loss should not be included in overall assessment of drug efficacy. Most objective studies have either been open[6,7] or placebo-controlled[8,9]. The only PGSI comparative study in dysfunctional uterine bleeding is that of Dockeray *et al.*[10] who have compared mefenamic acid and danazol in the treatment of established menorrhagia.

PATIENT SELECTION

While most studies are confined to patients with objective menorrhagia[6,7,9,10] (menstrual blood loss >80 ml), others[8] include all women with subjectively assessed excessive bleeding. Moreover, while most studies are based on clearly defined subject groups, e.g. unexplained excessive menstrual bleeding[6,7,9,10], others[8] include women who have undergone tubal ligation and patients with intrauterine devices, uterine fibroids or various bleeding diatheses.

STATISTICAL ANALYSIS

In most studies, treatment cycles have been compared with non-treatment or placebo-controlled cycles. Response to placebos may vary from 0% to 25% suggesting that emotional factors may be involved, although evidence for this has not been substantiated. Considerable variations in the efficacy of treatment may be achieved by comparing differences between mean and median values. The latter may be more appropriate as menstrual blood loss has a positively skewed distribution. Furthermore, individual volume reductions may differ markedly from individual percentage reductions. Likewise, mean (or median) volume reductions, expressed as a percentage, will differ from mean (or median) percentage reductions.

COEXISTING MENSTRUAL SYMPTOMS

Menorrhagia frequently coexists with dysmenorrhoea and other menstrual symptoms which may also require consideration if treatment is to be successful.

SIDE-EFFECTS AND PATIENT ACCEPTABILITY

While many women may accept treatment for two or three cycles during a trial, few are prepared to continue treatment indefinitely – especially if they have experienced adverse side-effects. Clinical trials should ideally give information on overall patient acceptability and long-term follow-up.

RESULTS OF OBJECTIVE STUDIES

The efficacy of mefenamic acid 500 mg, taken three times daily during menstruation, has been investigated in five studies[6-10] which have reported significant reductions in menstrual blood loss with menorrhagia due primarily to natural causes as opposed to intrauterine devices.

In the study of Anderson and co-workers[6] five patients with dysfunctional uterine bleeding were treated with mefenamic acid. Their mean pretreatment menstrual blood loss of 107 ml was reduced to 67 ml on treatment representing a reduction of 37.3% (8.8–57%).

Haynes *et al.*[7] studied 23 patients, one of whom dropped out due to severe diarrhoea. Median pretreatment menstrual blood loss of 137 ml was significantly reduced to 76 ml on treatment representing a 44.5%

reduction (p <0.001). Reduction in menstrual blood loss was achieved in 20 of the 22 patients but varied from 2% to 78%; and in two cases blood loss increased by 2% and 9%.

In the study of Fraser *et al.*[8] 69 patients, with a convincing history of excessive bleeding completed a double-blind, placebo-controlled trial. The study included six patients with intrauterine devices, two with fibroids, 25 tubal sterilizations and one with von Willebrand's disease. The overall mean menstrual blood loss during the placebo cycles was only 66.9 ml. Thirty patients (43%) had true menorrhagia (mean blood loss 100.8 ml), whereas 39 (57%) had menstrual blood losses of less than 80 ml (mean 45.8 ml). In 14 cases the loss was less than 35 ml. Overall, there was a significant mean reduction of 28.1% in menstrual blood loss between placebo- and mefenamic acid-treated cycles (p <0.001). For the 30 women with established menorrhagia the reduction was 30.3% with the greatest reduction recorded 80%. Significant reductions in blood loss (p <0.001) were seen in patients with ovulatory dysfunctional uterine bleeding and menorrhagia that developed after tubal ligation. There was also an indication, based on small sample sizes, that mefenamic acid reduced loss in women with anovulatory uterine bleeding, fibroids, intrauterine devices and von Willebrand's disease.

Muggeridge and Elder[9] studied 20 patients in a double-blind cross-over trial with placebo. There were five drop-outs including one patient who developed severe nausea, one with heavy bleeding leading to hysterectomy and another with irregular bleeding leading to hormone therapy. Mean menstrual loss was compared between two controlled cycles (182.4 ml), two placebo cycles (161.0 ml) and two treatment cycles (128.3 ml). Menstrual loss was decreased by treatment in 12 subjects while despite treatment it remained almost the same in one subject and increased in two subjects. The Wilcoxon test showed a significant reduction in menstrual loss of 29.7% in the treated cycles when compared with the control cycles (p <0.05), but there was no significant difference between treatment and placebo cycles.

Dockeray *et al.*[10] have undertaken an open parallel group randomized study comparing mefenamic acid and danazol. Menstrual loss was initially measured in two controlled cycles. During the second cycle an 8–10 ml menstrual blood sample was obtained through a uterine catheter on day 2 of menstruation for analysis of coagulation, fibrinolytic and prostaglandin activities (to be reported elsewhere). The volume of blood collected through the catheter was added to the volume estimated by the extraction process to calculate the total menstrual blood loss of the cycle. Twenty patients were treated with mefenamic acid. The results were based on 19 subjects as one woman with side-effects was withdrawn. The mean of the individual losses in the first two cycles (control cycles) was significantly higher than in the two treatment cycles (159.6 ml vs 127.3 ml), representing a 20% reduction (p <0.01, Mann–Whitney U-test).

Figure 1 illustrates the percentage changes in menstrual blood loss between the two control cycles and the two treatment cycles for each patient. The mean change was 22.3% on mefenamic acid (56% on danazol).

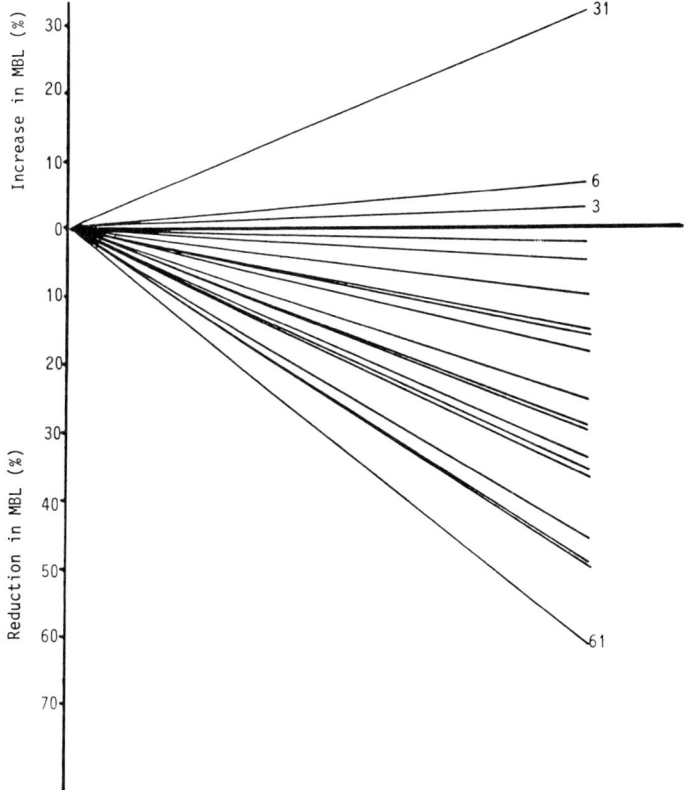

Figure 1 Mefenamic acid group (n = 19). Percentage change in menstrual blood loss between pretreatment cycles 1 and 2, and treatment cycles 3 and 4 (mean percentage change 22.3%)

Of the 130 patients who completed the five objective studies 91 had true menorrhagia. The overall mean percentage reduction was 31.9.

Haynes *et al.*[7] reported a highly significant correlation beween pretreatment menstrual blood loss and the average volume reduction in blood loss during therapy. Fraser and his colleagues[8] found the percentage reduction was generally greater in women with the highest placebo cycle loss. We found no relationship between individual percentage reductions and pretreatment blood loss although a positive correlation was found between volume reduction and pretreatment loss in 16 of 19 patients whose menstrual blood loss decreased on therapy.

DURATION OF MENSTRUATION

Mefenamic acid has been reported to have no effect on the duration of menstruation[7,10], although a highly significant reduction was found by Fraser and co-workers[8].

DYSMENORRHOEA AND OTHER MENSTRUAL SYMPTOMS

Mefenamic acid significantly improved pain scores in approximately 70% of patients with dysmenorrhoea associated with menorrhagia[8,10]. Fraser and his colleagues also reported a significant reduction in the duration of menstrually related headaches and diarrhoea but not in the number of days in nausea, vomiting, depression or breast tenderness[8].

SIDE-EFFECTS

The incidence of side-effects in the five objective studies ranged from nil (out of six patients) reported by Anderson and her co-workers[6] to 30%[10] where six out of 20 patients reported adverse effects. The most common events encountered were nausea, vomiting, abdominal discomfort, diarrhoea, headaches, dizziness and oedema.

PATIENT ACCEPTABILITY AND LONG-TERM FOLLOW-UP

In our study[10], nine of the 20 mefenamic acid-treated patients were unwilling to continue therapy because of inadequate reduction in menstrual blood loss. Two of these nine also suffered unacceptable side-effects. To date we have followed-up 22 patients treated with mefenamic acid with quantitatively proven menorrhagia (Dockeray, Sheppard and Bonnar, unpublished data), only seven patients (32%) considered mefenamic acid an acceptable form of treatment. Pretreatment menstrual blood loss of 112 ml (range 81–165 ml) was reduced to 77.3 ml, representing a reduction of 31%. Fraser and co-workers[14] followed 36 women who had experienced both a subjective and objective reduction in menstrual blood loss in their earlier trial[8]. Two women discontinued therapy because of drug-related dyspepsia but the menstrual blood losses were reduced from 65.6 ml in the earlier placebo cycles to 49.2 ml (25%) at 6–9 months and 42.8 ml (35%) at 12–15 months.

CONCLUSIONS

Mefenamic acid effectively reduces menstrual blood loss in approximately one-half of patients with subjectively assessed excessive bleeding, and in one-third of cases with objectively established menorrhagia. Long-term reductions in blood loss of approximately 25%–35% are generally confined to subjects with pretreatment losses of 60–160 ml. Overall patient acceptability is enhanced by the drug's beneficial effect on dysmenorrhoea and other menstrually related symptoms. Moreover, mefenamic acid need only be taken for 2–5 days each cycle thus avoiding any potentially serious complications from long-term use and cutting down prescribing costs.

REFERENCES

1. Guillebaud, J., Anderson, A.B.M. and Turnbull, A.C. (1978). Reduction by mefenamic acid of increased menstrual blood loss associated with intra-uterine contraception. *Br. J. Obstet. Gynaecol.*, **85**, 53–62
2. Davies, A.J., Anderson, A.B.M. and Turnbull, A.C. (1981). Reduction by

naproxen of excessive bleeding in women using intrauterine devices. *Obstet. Gynecol.*, **57**, 74–8

3. Rybo, G., Nilsson, S., Sikstrom, B. and Nygen, K.G. (1981). Naproxen in menorrhagia. *Lancet*, **i**, 608–9

4. Ylikorkala, O. and Viinikka, L. (1983). Comparison between antifibrinolytic and antiprostaglandin treatment in the reduction of increased menstrual blood loss in women with intrauterine contraceptive devices. *Br. J. Obstet. Gynaecol.*, **90**, 78–83

5. Mäkäräinen, L. and Ylikorkala, O. (1986). Ibuprofen prevents IUCD-induced increases in menstrual blood loss. *Br. J. Obstet. Gynaecol.*, **93**, 285–8

6. Anderson, A.B.M., Haynes, P.J., Guillebaud, J. and Turnbull, A.C. (1976). Reduction of menstrual loss by prostaglandin-synthetase inhibitors. *Lancet*, **i**, 774–6

7. Haynes, P.J., Flint, A.P., Guillebaud, J. and Turnbull, A.C. (1980). Studies in menorrhagia (a) Mefenamic acid, (b) Endometrial prostaglandin concentrations. *Int. J. Gynecol. Obstet.*, **17**, 567–72

8. Fraser, I.S., Pearse, C., Shearman, R.P., Elliott, P.M., McIlveen, J. and Markham, R. (1981). Efficiency of mefenamic acid in patients with a complaint of menorrhagia. *Obstet. Gynecol.*, **58**, 543–51

9. Muggeridge, J. and Elder, M.G. (1983). Mefenamic acid in the treatment of menorrhagia. *Res. Clin. Forums*, **5** (3), 83–8

10. Dockeray, C.J., Sheppard, B.L. and Bonnar, J. (1989). Comparison between mefenamic acid and danazol in the treatment of established menorrhagia. *Br. J. Obstet. Gynaecol.*, **96**, 840–4

11. Flower, R.J. and Vane, J.R. (1974). Inhibitions of prostaglandin synthesis. *Biochem. Pharmacol.*, **23**, 1439–50

12. Chan, W.Y. (1983). Prostaglandins and nonsteroidal anti-inflammatory drugs in dysmenorrhoea. *Ann. Rev. Pharmacol. Toxicol.*, **23**, 131–49

13. Rees, M.C.P., Canete-Soler, R., Bernal, A.L. and Turnbull, A.C. (1988). Effect of fenamates on prostaglandin E receptor binding. Preliminary communication. *Lancet*, 541–2

14. Fraser, I.S., McCarron, G., Markham, R., Robinson, M. and Smythe, E. (1983). Long term treatment of menorrhagia with mefenamic acid. *Obstet. Gynecol.*, **61**, 109–12

DISCUSSION

Dr M.C.P. Rees   Mr Dockeray's use of a uterine catheter might have confounded his results since an intrauterine catheter is known to affect endometrial blood flow.

Prof. R.W. Shaw May it not work in the other way, by stimulating prostaglandin production and reducing the loss?

Dr M.C.P. Rees It all depends on how much blood is sucked out, and this may be variable.

Mr. C.J. Dockeray Blood was not sucked out. But Prof. Shaw is quite right. There is a significant reduction in blood loss and the histogram for the Danol slide would have shown exactly the same thing. However, the catheter was only in for a short period of time and the overall result would be acceptable.

Dr M.C.P. Rees What should have been done is a control experiment, a couple of periods without a catheter and a couple of periods with a catheter to see if a catheter does have an effect on menstrual blood loss, as preliminary work before putting it in the middle of a drug study.

Prof. B.L. Sheppard In response to Dr Rees's comments, in fact what we did in that study was exactly what she suggested. We compared one control cycle without a catheter in and one control cycle with a catheter in, one treatment cycle with a catheter in and one treatment cycle without a catheter in. So they are comparable.

Dr H.M. Fraser I wanted to come back on the problem of dosage with mefenamic acid, we have found in general that we do not get such a good response with 250 mg TID, so we have consistently gone to 500 mg. We have a number of individual patients who require higher doses than that and their blood loss decreases as we give the higher doses.

Dr M.A. Lumsden In some cases a woman will get a better effect with mefenamic acid at a high dose, but this is not necessarily borne out with other synthetase inhibitors. For example with Naprosyn there have been studies which demonstrate that it is not a dose-related response.

Mr C.J. Dockeray We measured mefenamic acid levels in menstrual fluid and peripheral blood and found a correlation between response and drug level.

10

Danazol in dysfunctional uterine bleeding

R.W. Shaw

INTRODUCTION

The ideal medical treatment for the control of excessive menstrual blood loss in the absence of pelvic or other pathology has yet to be discovered. The commonest treatments utilized are cyclical hormone therapy, either progestogens alone or combined oestrogen/progestogen pills, prostaglandin synthetase inhibitors, or ethamsylate. Such treatments may be ineffective or have significant side-effects, or be contraindicated in women in their 40s in whom hormonal agents may be associated with an increased risk of thrombosis.

The vast majority of women with dysfunctional uterine bleeding have regular menstrual cycles with gonadotrophin and ovarian steroid hormone levels comparable to women with menstrual cycles in which there is normal menstrual blood loss[1]. In this Symposium the relevance of ovarian function in relationship to potential for the endometrium to synthesize various subgroups of prostaglandins and their relevance to control of menstrual blood loss has already been discussed (Chapters 1 and 2).

Anovulatory cycles and a lack of progesterone secretion may be highly relevant factors in potential genesis of dysfunctional uterine bleeding. However, all anovulatory cycles are not menorrhagic and indeed often quite the reverse. Progesterone/progestogen replacement therapy, i.e. luteal phase administration on days 16–25 might be expected to correct endometrial prostaglandin abnormalities in anovulatory cycles in patients with cystic glandular hyperplasia. However, the value of progestogen replacement therapy in subjects with dysfunctional uterine bleeding but regular ovulatory cycles is in question. Little quantitative data exist to support its use although progestogens are usually the first line of treatment in menorrhagia.

The administration of progestogens throughout the menstrual cycle (days 5–25 inclusive) is commonly adopted as an alternative treatment option in menorrhagia, but again with little objective menstrual blood loss measurement evidence of success. Here the treatment will induce poorly developed endometrium with attendant reduced menstrual blood loss following cessation of the progestogen course.

Danazol is an isoxazol derivative of 17α-ethinyl-testosterone. It is known to have a number of effects on the hypothalamic pituitary ovarian axis. Administration of danazol in the menstrual cycle induces alteration in pulsatile gonadotrophin release and inhibition of the midcycle gonadotrophin surge. These result in inhibition of normal follicular maturation and growth and a suppression of oestradiol-17β production. These effects are to some extent dose-related and at high doses a hypo-oestrogenic and hypoprogestogenic environment develops. The endometrium on prolonged danazol therapy is likely to be atrophic[2]. In addition, danazol has been shown to inhibit ovarian and adrenal steroidogenesis directly in some species[3,4].

All these above effects of danazol might be beneficial in treating patients with dysfunctional uterine bleeding, and indeed it has been investigated in such a role. The first publication evaluating the efficacy of danazol in patients with menorrhagia, was published by Chimbira *et al.* in 1979[5]. In this study the patients were given a dose of 400 mg danazol daily for a 12-week treatment period and objective menstrual blood loss assessments were performed. These indicated that during the 1st month of treatment there was a reduction in objective menstrual blood loss of 41.5% and this was increased to 90.7% after 3 months of treatment. Many of the subjects becoming amenorrhoeic during the second and third cycles of therapy.

MODE OF ACTION OF DANAZOL IN DYSFUNCTIONAL UTERINE BLEEDING

As indicated above the endometrium in women on danazol therapy is atrophic. This could be associated with reduced circulating levels of oestradiol, found by some workers[6], although not by others[7]. Effects of danazol administration on steroid hormone concentrations in women with menorrhagia were studied at great length by Chimbira *et al.*[8]. This was a study of 13 patients who received 400 mg danazol daily for 12 weeks with serial measurements of serum oestradiol and progesterone throughout treatment. Serum progesterone levels remained below the levels of detection of the assay (at less than 3 nmol/l) throughout treatment whilst serum oestradiol-17β fell progressively during the first 2 to 3 weeks of treatment and them remained at less than 100 pmol/l thereafterwards (see Figure 1). Many of these subjects became amenorrhoeic, but no direct correlation could be found between the circulating oestradiol-17β level 1 week before menstrual bleeding and the volume of blood loss when assessed during the 2nd and 3rd months of treatment (see Figure 2). There was a wide variation between the levels of circulating oestradiol-17β achieved in these individuals and no correlation was found between the level of oestradiol-17β, amount of blood loss seen or the development of amenorrhoea in this group of subjects with previous established menorrhagia (>80 ml measured menstrual blood loss per cycle). In some patients oestradiol levels were similar to those found in postmenopausal patients, and indeed some patients did report occurrence of hot flushes. In some subjects who were studied with daily blood samples prior to the onset of bleeding, there was no evidence of a fall in oestradiol occurring to initiate the onset of bleeding.

On the other hand danazol has been shown to have direct effects on myometrial and endometrial receptors for oestradiol and progesterone[9] and these may interfere with endometrial growth responses to circulating steroid hormone levels and tissue growth factors.

Another mechanism by which danazol may have an effect is through alteration in the endometrium's ability to synthesize prostaglandins. However, this ability appears to be unchanged as judged by the data published on endometrial prostaglandin synthesis in subjects receiving danazol as reported by Cameron *et al*[10].

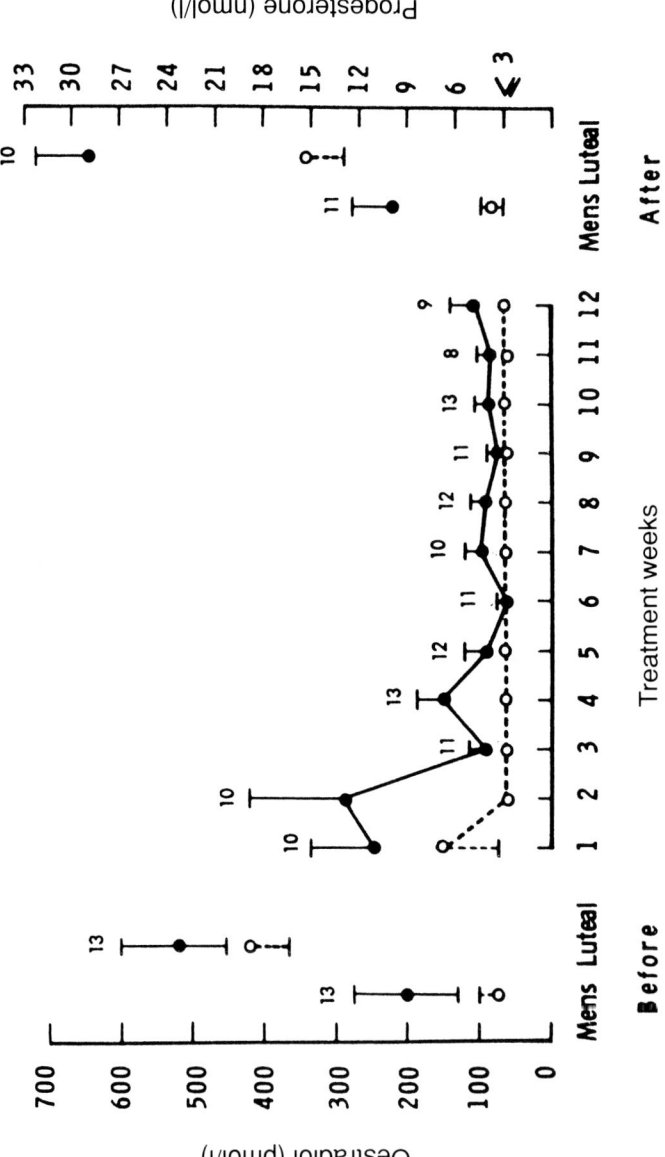

Figure 1 Serum oestradiol and progesterone values in patients receiving 400 mg danazol daily for the treatment of dysfunctional uterine bleeding. (From Chimbira *et al.*, 1980[8], with permission)

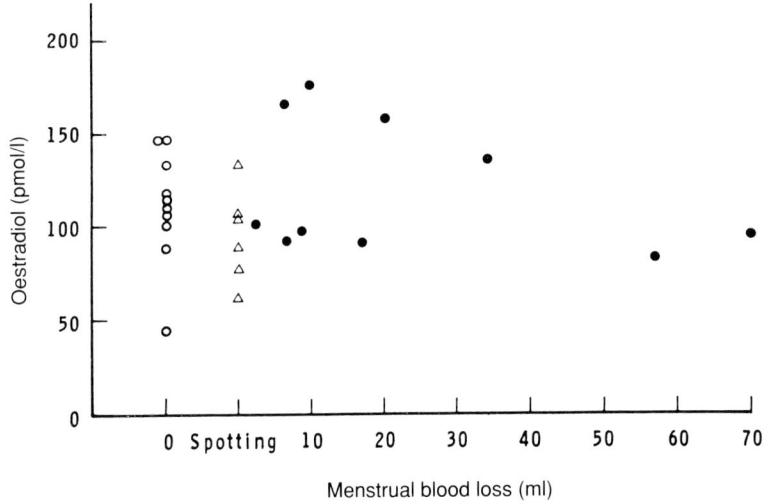

Figure 2 Lack of correlation between circulating oestradiol-17β levels and amount of menstrual blood loss in patients receiving danazol. (From Chimbira *et al.*, 1980[8] with permission)

Our own unpublished data indicate that doses of 200 mg danazol daily over 3 months, lead to a reduction in uterine size, established by measurement of uterine volume using ultrasound and also a reduction in endometrial thickness as measured by ultrasound (see Chapter 5). These data seem to indicate a direct effect of danazol on endometrial mass *per se* which may be one mechanism in the mode of action of improvement in reducing measured menstrual blood loss in subjects receiving danazol.

UNCONTROLLED STUDIES USING DANAZOL

The effectiveness of danazol at 400 mg daily was first reported by Chimbira *et al.*[5] and further confirmed in a single-blind placebo-controlled trial of eight patients receiving one placebo capsule daily for two cycles and then 200 mg danazol daily for two cycles, during which menstrual blood losses were objectively measured[11]. Placebo therapy did not significantly alter menstrual blood loss but danazol treatment significantly reduced the menstrual blood loss in the first treatment cycle to 50 ± 9 ml, with a further greater reduction seen during the second cycle (10 ± 7 ml) and in the third cycle (13 ± 8 ml). Several women collected menstrual pads from post-treatment cycles and in the five studied, menstrual blood loss had increased again to a mean of 100 ± 28 ml by the 3rd post-treatment month[11].

The same authors then compared a dose of danazol of 200 mg daily with a dose of 100 mg daily and its effects on measured menstrual blood loss are shown in Figure 3. This figure also has the data from their previous reported study in 1979 with a dose of 400 mg daily[5]. It was found that in the first cycle on 200 mg daily, menstrual blood loss was not significantly reduced but thereafter there was a significant reduction compared with the pretreatment mean. Whilst one patient on 200 mg daily had complete amenorrhoea from the commencement of treatment and another patient had only one episode of bleeding during the 12 weeks of therapy, the majority of subjects continued to menstruate and there was no significant change in the cycle length. The duration of days of bleeding however was significantly reduced from a mean of 6.8 ± 0.7 pretreatment to 4.1 ± 0.6 in the second and third treatment cycles.

In subjects on 100 mg daily, of the 16 patients treated one had amenorrhoea in the 2nd treatment month and one in the 3rd treatment month, but five patients had four episodes of vaginal bleeding during the 12 weeks of danazol therapy. On 100 mg the mean menstrual blood loss of patients treated was reduced to within the normal range although to a lesser degree than either 200 mg or 400 mg. With 100 mg daily a shortened cycle length in some patients was noted and there was no significant effect of danazol 100 mg daily on the duration of bleeding[11]. In a more recent study Fraser[12] using a subjective record for blood loss assessment, utilized dosages of danazol between 200 mg and 800 mg daily for up to 6 months treatment. He confirmed that with higher doses of danazol the majority of patients became amenorrhoeic whilst at lower doses they continued to menstruate regularly although the menstrual blood loss was significantly reduced.

Both Fraser[12] and Chimbira *et al.*[11] found that the increased menstrual bleeding had relapsed between 3 and 6 months after ceasing active therapy and the majority of subjects required or sought further active treatment. From these studies it was shown that danazol at 200 mg daily was also significant in reducing menstrual blood loss in objectively proven menorrhagia. Blood loss was not seen to be significantly reduced by placebo therapy in the findings of others[13] and this supports the view that

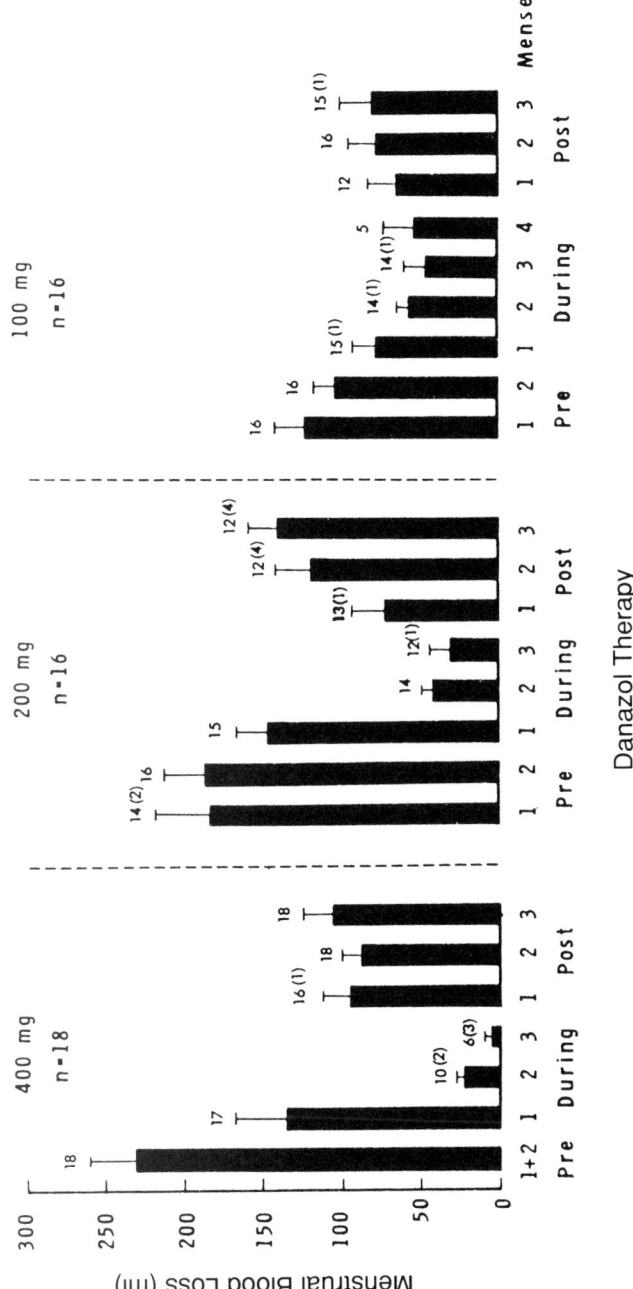

Figure 3 Effect of danazol therapy at various doses on amount of measured menstrual blood loss in patients with menorrhagia. (From Chimbira *et al.*, 1980[11] with permission)

reassurance alone will not suppress menstrual blood loss in women with dysfunctional uterine bleeding.

RANDOMIZED COMPARATIVE STUDIES USING DANAZOL

Several randomized comparative studies have now been reported and all confirm danazol's effectiveness for the treatment of dysfunctional uterine bleeding, when compared with other agents.

In a comparative study of measured blood loss assessments Cameron *et al.*[10] found a reduction in mean percentage blood loss of 74.9% on danazol 200 mg, whilst a reduction of only 16% in measured blood loss was achieved with norethisterone 10 mg daily from days 15 to 26 of the cycle.

In our own comparative trial comparing subjects with dysfunctional uterine bleeding with blood loss measured using alkaline haematin dilution technique[14], all subjects had measured blood loss in excess of a mean of 80 ml over two assessment cycles. Pathology was excluded by D & C or vabra curettage plus pelvic ultrasound prior to treatment. Patients were then run in with placebo capsules which were followed by three treatment cycles of active therapy, receiving either norethisterone 15 mg daily from days 19 to 26 of the cycle or danazol 200 mg daily throughout the cycle. All subjects had been established as having ovulatory dysfunctional uterine bleeding. The initial data from this ongoing study have been tabulated in Table 1. It will be seen that few of the patients receiving norethisterone showed consistent reduction of menstrual blood loss to less than 80 ml per cycle. Treatment with norethisterone however was well tolerated and patients had regular cycles with few episodes of breakthrough bleeding.

Patients receiving danazol in the 2nd and 3rd month of treatment in the majority of instances had a reduction of menstrual blood loss to less than 80 ml per cycle. In two individuals there appeared to be no response and on further investigation of these subjects to exclude unsuspected pelvic pathology, no abnormalities were found. In many of the individuals recieving Danol, there was a tendency for alteration in cycle length with a shortening of the cycle.

Table 1 Measured menstrual blood losses, mean of two control cycles on placebo and during treatment following randomization

Norethisterone (15 mg daily day 19–26)			Danazol (200 mg daily)		
Baseline (Mean of two)	*Month 1*	*Month 3*	*Baseline (Mean of two)*	*Month 1*	*Month 3*
176	170	234	181	93	15
223	180	208	260	298	397
103	68	139	86	39	56
189	79	97	235	198	309
395	287	329	137	43	22
155	185	175	99	<10	Nil
168	300	189	156	110	82
81	67	82			
112	74	102			

SIDE-EFFECTS WITH DANAZOL

Much has been written on the side-effects of danazol in women being treated for endometriosis in which disease often high doses between 400 and 800 mg daily may be utilized to achieve therapeutic effects. Some side-effects, particularly weight gain, are commonly seen, as are tiredness, skeletal pain, headaches and irritability. The tendency is for these problems to be dose-related and this is confirmed by the study of Chimbira *et al.*[11] in menorrhagia patients – the data are summarized in Table 2. To reduce the incidence of side-effects of danazol, dosage should be kept at the lowest effective dose and regimes using a reducing dose of danazol need to be investigated for their effect in controlling dysfunctional uterine bleeding.

CONCLUSION

In summary, danazol at 200 mg daily will significantly reduce menstrual blood loss when administered for at least 3 months. In some patients a dose of 400 mg daily may be necessary. Although danazol at a dose of

Table 2 Side-effects observed in patients received danazol for 12 weeks to treat menorrhagia. (Adapted from Chimbira *et al.* 1980[11])

	Daily dose of danazol (mg)		
	100 *(n=16)*	*200* *(n=16)*	*400* *(n=18)*
Mean weight gain (kg)	2.1	2.3	4.5
Tiredness/sleepiness	6	5	7
Musculoskeletal pain	2	4	7
Headaches	5	6	5
Skin rashes	2	3	6
Irritability	1	3	4

200 mg daily is more expensive than other medical treatments, it undoubtedly leads to the most significant reduction in measured menstrual blood loss. A further advantage of danazol is the carry-over effect on cessation of treatment which may persist for two or three post-treatment cycles.

With a dose of 200 mg daily some might allude to a higher incidence of side-effects than seen with other medications used in the treatment of dysfunctional uterine bleeding but direct comparisons have never been made appropriately. A decision to use danazol in dysfunctional uterine bleeding in patients who complain of dysmenorrhoea in addition, is also advantageous since both symptoms can be helped. Lack of effect of danazol on the coagulation system[5] makes it a safe alternative to other synthetic steroids in women over the age of 40, thus making danazol a useful addition to the now wide range of drugs used in an attempt to treat unexplained menorrhagia.

REFERENCES

1. Haynes, P.J., Anderson, A.B.M. and Turnbull, A.C. (1979). Patterns of menstrual blood loss in menorrhagia. *Res. Clin. Forums*, **1**, 73–8
2. Greenblatt, R.B., Dmowski, W.P., Mahesh, V.B. and Scholer, H.F.L.

(1971). Clinical studies with an antigonadotrophin danazol. *Fertil. Steril.*, **22**, 102–12

3. Barbieri, R.L., Canick, J.A., Makris, A., Todd, R.B., Davies, J.I. and Ryan, K.J. (1977). Danazol inhibits steroidogenesis. *Fertil. Steril.*, **28**, 809–13

4. Tsang, B.K., Henderson, K.M. and Armstrong, D.T. (1979). Effect of danazol on estradiol–17B and progesterone secretion by porcine ovarian cells *in vitro*. *Am. J. Obstet. Gynecol.*, **133**, 256–9

5. Chimbira, T.H., Cope, E., Anderson, A.B.M. and Bolton, F.G. (1979). The effect of danazol on menorrhagia, coagulation mechanisms, haematological indices and body weight. *Br. J. Obstet. Gynaecol.*, **86**, 46–50

6. Wood, G.P., Wu, G.H., Flickinger, G.L. and Mikhail, G. (1975). Hormonal changes associated with danazol therapy. *Obstet. Gynecol.*, **45**, 302–4

7. Andrews, M.C. and Wentz, A.C. (1975). The effects of danazol on gonadotrophins and steroid blood levels in normal and anovulatory women. *Am. J. Obstet. Gynecol.*, **121**, 817–28

8. Chimbira, T.H., Anderson, A.B.M., Cope, E. and Turnbull, A.C. (1980). Effect of danazol on serum gonadotrophins and steroid hormone concentration in women with menorrhagia. *Br. J. Obstet. Gynaecol.*, **87**, 330–6

9. Tamaya, T., Furata, M., Motoyama, T., Boku, S., Okowo, Y. and Okada, H. (1978). Mechanisms of antiprogestational action of synthetic steroids. *Acta Endocrinol. (Kbh)*, **88**, 190–8

10. Cameron, I.T., Leask, R., Kelly, R.W. and Baird, D.T. (1987). The effects of danazol and mefenamic acid, norethisterone and a progesterone – impregnated coil on endometrial prostaglandin concentrations in women with menorrhagia. *Prostaglandins*, **34**, 99–100

11. Chimbira, T.H., Anderson, A.B.M., Naise, C., Cope, E. and Turnbull, A.C. (1980). Reduction of menstrual blood loss by danazol in unexplained menorrhagia: lack of effect of placebo. *Br. J. Obstet. Gynaecol.*, **25**, 224–6

12. Fraser, I.S. (1985). Treatment of dysfunctional uterine bleeding with danazol. *Aust. N.Z. J. Obstet. Gynaecol.*, **25**, 224–6

13. Harrison, R.F. and Campbell, S. (1976). A double-blind trial of ethamsylate in the treatment of primary and intrauterine-device menorrhagia. *Lancet*, **2**, 283–5

14. Hallberg, L. and Nilsson, L. (1964). Determination of menstrual blood loss. *Scand. J. Clin. Lab. Invest.*, **16**, 244–8

DISCUSSION

Mr C.J. Dockeray   There was a question as regards danazol. I understood from Professor Shaw's presentation that there was very little in the way of side-effects?

Prof. R.W. Shaw   At 200 mg/day that is correct in terms of serious side-effects.

Mr C.J. Dockeray   Yet Dr Gardner suggested that some patients were not prepared to continue the drug in her study (see Chapter 12). In our own study 75% had side-effects at 200 mg/day and some of these patients had breast atrophy.

It is also very important to warn patients that they may get hirsutism or hoarseness, because if they do treatment should be discontinued immediately.

Taking that situation, coupled with the fact that their menorrhagia will be back to square one after 3 months, I would very much query whether danazol has any role to play in the treatment of menorrhagia.

Prof. R.W. Shaw   The doses used by Dr Gardner were 600 mg/day, and so we are talking of a very different dosage and one would expect to get a much higher incidence of side-effect profiles as it is dose related.

With regard to that last statement, all I can point out from the studies is that danazol is effective at reducing blood loss. Of course one has to be careful in its use in terms of contraceptive protection in all cycles at a dose of 200 mg/day.

But the other aspects relate to how all patients should be counselled no matter what the therapy. We have to discuss with them possible side-effects and the relevance of them, and presentation back, should they develop

Any other treatment that we have looked at is less effective, other than LHRH analogues, at inhibiting blood loss to the same degree, so one has to bear that in relationship to the problems which are inherent in the compound.

I would not advocate it as the first-line treatment, but in patients who have tried other methods of therapy which have not been effective then this is a drug which could be useful.

11

Treatment of dysfunctional uterine bleeding with oral, intramuscular or intrauterine progestogens

I.S. Fraser

INTRODUCTION

Dysfunctional uterine bleeding has been defined as excessive bleeding (heavy, prolonged or frequent) of uterine origin, which is not due to organic pelvic disease or a systemic condition[1]. It is convenient to divide patients into those with predominantly anovulatory or predominantly ovulatory dysfunctional uterine bleeding. This has particular importance in relation to treatment with oral progestogens. This paper will be concerned mainly with patients who have chronic dysfunctional uterine bleeding, although anecdote suggests that high-dose oral progestogens alone may have an occasional role in the management of an acute episode of excessively heavy bleeding.

A clinical diagnosis of anovulatory dysfunctional uterine bleeding may often be made with reasonable accuracy on history alone, taking into account the patient's age and cycle regularity, but for research purposes this should be confirmed by progesterone measurements or endometrial biopsy. It should also be borne in mind that few patients at the extremes of reproductive age are consistently anovulatory or ovulatory[2-4].

RATIONALE FOR USING PROGESTOGENS

Progestogens are molecules which bind to the progesterone receptor, and stimulate some of the hormonal actions of progesterone[5]. The classical biological action on which their activity is based is the maintenance of pregnancy in animals in which the corpus luteum has been removed. In the context of the present paper, their actions on the endometrium are of particular importance.

Secretory transformation of the endometrium

Progestogens will induce a series of biochemical and morphological changes, called secretory transformation, within an endometrium which has previously been primed by exposure to oestrogen alone. Optimal secretory change seems to follow 10–14 days of oestrogen exposure – the average duration of the normal follicular phase. The relative dosage and duration of exposures to oestrogen and progestogen are important in determining the extent of secretory change, and different progestogens appear to have different qualititative effects[6].

Inhibition of endometrial proliferation

One of the actions of progestogens within endometrium is to inhibit the proliferative effect of oestrogen administered simultaneously. Thus progestogen exposure from early in the menstrual cycle will result in a much thinner endometrium than normal – as seen with modern combined oral contraceptives[7]. This usually results in less blood loss at the next menstruation/withdrawal bleed[8].

Endometrial suppression/atrophy

Continued long-term exposure of endometrium to progestogens results in inhibition or suppression of secretory change, and the end-result of this is a histological appearance which is indistinguishable from atrophy[9]. What appears to happen is that continued progestogen exposure prevents

140

regeneration of progestogen and oestrogen receptors, hence preventing any biological expression of these two hormones. This unresponsive tissue gradually becomes thinner and much less active, although initiallly there is pronounced stromal decidual change even after disappearance of glandular secretory activity[9,10]. Bleeding is much less likely from this endometrium, and most women will develop amenorrhoea[11]. However, some women with this type of exposure will experience erratic episodes of unpredictable scanty bleeding.

Inhibition of follicular growth and ovulation

Exposure to continuous high-dose progestogen will effectively prevent follicular growth and the endogenous secretion of follicular phase patterns of oestradiol[12]. This will contribute to the maintenance of a thin endometrium, which is less likely to bleed heavily.

ADMINISTRATION OF PROGESTOGENS

Progestogens may be administered by almost any route, including oral, intramuscular, subcutaneous, vaginal, rectal, intrauterine or transdermal, although, in practice, high enough endometrial levels for treatment of dysfunctional uterine bleeding can only be achieved by oral, intramuscular or intrauterine routes. These will be considered in detail.

Oral progestogens

It is logical, and anecdotally effective, to treat *anovulatory* women with cyclical oral progestogens, but little objective information is available[13,14]. The use of oral progestogens to treat *ovulatory* dysfunctional uterine bleeding is often reasonable, but results can be disappointing because of failure to use an appropriate regimen.

Oral progestogens can be used in four broadly different regimens for the management of chronic dysfunctional uterine bleeding:

(1) Day 16–25, luteal replacement or supplementation (secretory transformation);

(2) Day 5–25, reduced endometrial growth (inhibition of endometrial proliferation and inhibition of follicle growth);
(3) Continuous, endometrial suppression (atrophy/amenorrhoea);
(4) Combination oral contraceptives.

Replacement of absent endogenous progesterone by luteal phase oral progestogens in the anovulatory patient makes good clinical sense, but there are no good clinical studies to confirm this. We have limited data indicating a substantial and progressive reduction in measured menstrual blood loss in six women with anovulatory dysfunctional uterine bleeding treated with oral norethisterone (NET) or medroxyprogesterone acetate (MPA) three times daily for 14 days each cycle (Fraser, unpublished data). Menstrual blood loss was reduced from 131 ml before treatment to 80 ml and 64 ml in the first two treatment cycles respectively. In those women with endometrial cystic glandular hyperplasia, or with particularly high circulating oestrogen levels, higher or more prolonged dosage may be required. Usually dosages of NET of 5 mg bd or tds, or MPA 10 mg bd or tds are required.

Treatment of women with ovulatory dysfunctional uterine bleeding (and normal circulating progesterone levels) using luteal phase oral progestogen supplementation seems illogical, although it is widely used in clinical practice. Early subjective studies suggested that it might be effective in many ovulatory women[13]. Limited objective data confirm that this treatment is of little value[15]. Cameron et al.[15] found a non-significant reduction in measured menstrual blood loss from 131 to 110 ml in six women with ovulatory dysfunctional uterine bleeding treated with 10 days of luteal norethisterone 5 mg bd. Use of oral progestogens for 21 days out of 28 may be more logical and we have demonstrated some objective benefit in seven out of 10 ovulatory women (Fraser, unpublished data). Measured blood loss in the whole group was reduced from a pretreatment level of 112 ml to 76 ml in the first treatment cycle and 71 ml in the second. Three women exhibited dramatic reductions in blood loss, four were moderately improved and three showed little or no change.

Many women with ovulatory dysfunctional uterine bleeding will also obtain substantial benefit from complete suppression of menstruation using continuous oral progestogen, although some will experience occasional breakthrough bleeding on this regimen. Combination oestrogen–progestogen oral contraceptives, especially those with higher progestogen dosages, will significantly reduce bleeding in many with ovulatory dysfunctional uterine bleeding[8].

The disadvantages of long-term moderate and high-dose oral progestogens have been given little attention, but they are nevertheless of considerable importance in view of the potentially protracted nature of dysfunctional uterine bleeding treatment. Much of the detailed information on these aspects comes from studies of depot medroxy-progesterone acetate (DMPA) used as a contraceptive[16]. Reported side-effects, which may be troublesome with high-dose oral use, include weight gain, nausea, bloating, ankle oedema, headaches, depression and other mood changes, loss of libido, acne, hirsutism and breakthrough bleeding. Concerns have been expressed about possible long-term metabolic effects including minor changes in carbohydrate tolerance and circulating lipids. It is possible that these may lead to an increase in the risk of hypertension and cardiovascular disease, in a similar manner to combination oral contraceptives[17]. In theory, the risk could be expected to be less than with combined oral contraceptives, since progestogens have little or no adverse effect on the coagulation system. However, data on risk are not available. In view of the situation with oral contraceptives[18], attention should also be paid to the possibility of a very small increase in risk of breast and cervical cancer – and benign liver tumours – with prolonged use (although this is still far from clear with oral contraceptives). It can be expected that progestogens will have other therapeutic benefits, such as reductions in risk of endometrial and ovarian cancer, pelvic inflammatory disease, benign breast disease, etc.

Intramuscular progestogens

It has been suggested that DMPA may be a suitable therapy for dysfunctional uterine bleeding because it induces amenorrhoea in about 50% of women by 1 year of use[11], but the 15%–20% incidence of episodes of frequent or prolonged bleeding make this treatment unacceptable to many.

Intrauterine progestogens

Intrauterine release of progesterone[15,19,20] or levonorgestrel (Andersson and Rybo, unpublished data) from third generation intrauterine devices results in dramatic suppression of menstrual blood loss in women with menorrhagia. This therapeutic approach results in high local concentrations of progestogen in the endometrium, but relatively little systemic absorption. Andersson and Rybo have demonstrated in 20 women a mean 86% reduction in measured blood loss after 3 months and 97% reduction after 12 months use of an intrauterine device releasing 20 µg levonorgestrel per day. In addition, it is a highly effective contraceptive which has a duration of action in excess of 5 years[21].

The major disadvantage of this route of administration is the occurrence of nuisance-value spotting or intermenstrual bleeding during the first few months. This is much worse with the progesterone-releasing intrauterine device than with the levonorgestrel version. Some women develop amenorrhoea with continued treatment, although ovulation is usually unaffected. There is no evidence of long-term adverse effects of endometrial exposure to progestogens, and with this approach systemic metabolic effects should be minimal. Hence, this may become a very important approach to the long-term hormonal management of ovulatory and anovulatory dysfunctional uterine bleeding in the future.

SUPERVISION OF THERAPY

Consideration should be given to the manner of clinical supervision, and to the need for more frequent or more thorough supervision in women with risk factors for treatment. Patients should be seen 3-monthly initially for review of therapy, side-effects and blood pressure, and this assessment may usefully include a menstrual calendar. Thereafter, patients should be seen 6–12-monthly, with an annual examination of blood pressure, breasts, abdomen and pelvis (including cervical smear). Haematological and biochemical assessments, and mammograms, should be carried out as indicated.

CONCLUSION

For over 30 years progestogens have been used in the treatment of dysfunctional uterine bleeding, yet objective evidence for their efficacy is scanty. There are limited data to support the use of oral progestogens given as luteal progestational replacement in anovulatory patients, and as more prolonged (3 weeks out of 4, or continuous) regimens in ovulatory patients. In those women who respond well, therapy may need to be continued for many months or years, hence potential side-effects or complications of therapy should be taken into account. Increasing evidence suggests that the new progestogen-releasing intrauterine devices may prove to be an extremely valuable option for the treatment of dysfunctional uterine bleeding.

REFERENCES

1. Fraser, I.S. (1985). The dysfunctional uterus – dysmenorrhoea and dysfunctional uterine bleeding. In Shearman, R.P. (ed.). *Clinical Reproductive Endocrinology*, pp. 579–98 (Edinburgh: Churchill-Livingstone)
2. Southam, A.L. (1959). The natural history of menstrual disorders. *Ann. N. Y. Acad. Sci.*, **75**, 840–54
3. Collett, M.E., Wertenberger, G.E. and Fiske, V.M. (1954). The effect of age upon the pattern of the menstrual cycle. *Fertil. Steril.*, **5**, 437–48
4. Fraser, I.S. and Baird, D.T. (1974). Blood production and ovarian secretion rates of estradiol-17β and estrone in women with dysfunctional uterine bleeding. *J. Clin. Endocrinol. Metab.*, **39**, 564–70
5. Rozenbaum, H. (1982). Relationships between chemical structure and biological properties of progestogens. *Am. J. Obstet. Gynecol.*, **142**, 719–24
6. Whitehead, M.I., Townsend, P.T., Pryse-Davies, J., Ryder, T.A. and King, R.J.B. (1981). Effects of estrogens and progestins on the biochemistry and morphology of the post-menopausal endometrium. *N. Engl. J. Med.*, **305**, 1599–605
7. Ober, W.B. (1977). Effects of oral and intrauterine administration of contraceptives on the uterus. *Hum. Pathol.*, **8**, 513–27
8. Nilsson, L. and Rybo, G. (1971). Treatment of menorrhagia. *Am. J. Obstet. Gynecol.*, **110**, 713–20
9. Khoo, S.K., Mackay, E.V. and Adam, R.R. (1971). Contraception with a six-monthly injection of progestogen: 3. Effects on the endometrium. *Aust. N. Z. J. Obstet. Gynaecol.*, **11**, 226–32

145

10. Roberts, D.K., Morbelt, D.V. and Powell, L.C. (1975). The ultrastructural response of human endometrium to medroxyprogesterone acetate. *Am. J. Obstet. Gynecol.*, **123**, 811–18

11. Odlind, V. and Fraser, I.S. (1989). Hormonal contraception and menstrual bleeding disturbances: a clinical overview. In D'Arcangues, C., Fraser, I.S., Newton, J.R. and Odlind, V. (eds). *Contraception and Mechanisms of Endometrial Bleeding*. (Cambridge: Cambridge University Press) (in press)

12. Jeppsson, S., Gershagen, S., Johansson, E.D.B. and Rannevik, G. (1982). Plasma levels of medroxyprogesterone acetate (MPA), sex hormone-binding globulin, gonadal steroids, gonadotrophins and prolactin in women during long-term use of DMPA (Depo-Provera) as a contraceptive. *Acta Endocrinol.*, **99**, 339–43

13. Bishop, P.M.F. and de Almeida, J.C.C. (1960). Treatment of functional menstrual disorders with norethisterone. *Br. Med. J.*, **1**, 1103–12

14. Hoffman, D.I., Lobo, R.A. and Mishell, D.R., Jr (1985). Treatment of dysfunctional uterine bleeding. In Baird, D.T. and Michie, E.A. (eds). *Mechanism of Menstrual Bleeding*, pp. 253–62 Serono Symposia Publications, Volume 25. (New York: Raven Press)

15. Cameron, I.T., Leask, R., Kelly, R.W. and Baird, D.T. (1987). The effects of danazol, mefenamic acid, norethisterone and a progesterone-impregnated coil on endometrial prostaglandin concentrations in women with menorrhagia. *Prostaglandins*, **34**, 99–110

16. Fraser, I.S. and Weisberg, E. (1981). A comprehensive review of injectable contraception with special emphasis on depot medroxyprogesterone acetate. *Med. J. Aust.*, Supplement, **1**, 1–19

17. Drife, J. (1989). Complications of combined oral contraception. In Filshie, M. and Guillebaud, J. (eds). *Contraception: Science and Practice*, pp. 39–51. (London: Butterworths)

18. Vessey, M.P. (1989). Oral contraception and cancer. In Filshie, M. and Guillebaud, J. (eds). *Contraception: Science and Practice*, pp. 52–68. (London: Butterworths)

19. Newton, J.R., Snowden, S.A. and Parsons, V. (1976). Control of menstrual bleeding during haemodialysis. *Br. Med. J.*, **1**, 1016–17

20. Bergkvist, A. and Rybo, G. (1983). Treatment of menorrhagia with intra-uterine release of progesterone. *Br. J. Obstet. Gynaecol.*, **90**, 255–8

21. Luukkainen, T., Allonen, H., Haukkamaa, M., Lahteenmaki, P., Nilsson, C.G. and Toivonen, J. (1986). Five years experience with levonorgestrel-releasing intrauterine devices. *Contraception*, **33**, 139–48

DISCUSSION

Dr M.A. Lumsden   When the patients went on to norethisterone for 21 days, was there any increase in side-effects and what proportion wanted to carry on with the treatment?

Prof. I.S. Fraser   This was a slightly biased group in that they were mostly treatment failures from one of the prostaglandin inhibitors, and the majority of the ovulatory cases (six) were happy to continue thereafter.
Side-effects were minor and of nuisance value.

Dr A.J. Gordon   I find progesterones useful in women with a short cycle length, where at least we can try to get them back to a 28-day cycle. But are they in Australia leading the way in the sense that they are using much more medroxyprogesterone acetate than we are? I seem to get the impression that it is perhaps safer to use in terms of its effects on high and low density lipoprotein levels.

Prof. I.S. Fraser   It is a moot point as to which progestogen is best, and the arguments can be looked at from a number of points of view. Malcolm Whitehead's data suggests that norethisterone probably has a more specific, and perhaps slightly better effect on the endometrium; admittedly that is in postmenopausal hormone replacement and high doses of medroxyprogesterone acetate would be needed.
Nobody has really done large enough, good enough long-term metabolic studies comparing equipotent or clinically equally potent doses of different progestogens and so we use them interchangeably. I think medroxyprogesterone acetate is a good progestogen. I tend to use it as my first choice but I do not have anything specific against norethisterone.

Dr D.R. Abramovich   If patients are to be treated with progestogens or the prostaglandin inhibitors, would a greater success be obtained if they were hysteroscoped first, in view of the evidence that has been put forward that there are undiagnosable intrauterine problems?

Prof. I.S. Fraser   Yes. I would advocate hysteroscopy. There are now ample studies in the literature showing that blind curettage misses a lot. Hysteroscopy picks up a considerable number of unsuspected cases of intrauterine pathology.

Mefenamic acid does not work very well with fibroids; the occasional one responds. Patients with adenomyosis, endometriosis and menorrhagia do seem to respond reasonably well. Whether those are conditions that coexist with their dysfunctional bleeding or whether they are causing the problem I do not know, but some of those respond to mefenamic acid, and so mefenamic acid is worth a try.

Mr E. Versi We have been talking about the use of gestogens in dysfunctional uterine bleeding and we have discussed how it has to be for the long term and at reasonably high doses. It strikes me that there might be a negative effect on the HDL to LDL ratio and that there may be a long-term negative effect on the cardiovascular system. Is there any data on this and is there any work on the newer generation progestogens?

Prof. I.S. Fraser The simple answers are no and no. It is very sad, but in this area we have relatively little long-term data on any of the therapeutic agents that we use.

There is relatively little metabolic data even on the progestogen regimens that we use in the short term and that needs to be addressed as a matter of urgency.

But I agree entirely. I do have my reservations about potential metabolic hazards from long-term use of a number of these agents. We have touched on danazol, which certainly does alter HDL cholesterol downward substantially and they need to be looked at.

In terms of the newer progestogens, I am not aware of any data in their use for gynaecological reasons.

Prof. B.L. Sheppard Those menstrual blood loss results Professor Fraser showed with the levonorgestrel device were impressive, but one of the other side-effects of the progestosert was the increase in ectopic pregnancy rate. Was that a problem with the levonorgestrel device?

Prof. I.S. Fraser No. It does not appear to be a problem.

12

LHRH analogues in the treatment of menorrhagia

R. Gardner and R.W. Shaw

In the absence of pelvic or general medical pathology there is as yet no ideal medical treatment for women with menorrhagia, which still remains one of the commonest gynaecological disorders presenting at the out-patient clinic. The response of the individual to the different available treatments is variable and most frequently offers only temporary relief of symptoms while treatment continues. The search for alternative drugs to treat this benign yet debilitating condition has led to an interest in the luteinizing hormone-releasing hormone (LHRH) analogues.

MODE OF ACTION OF LHRH ANALOGUES

LHRH analogues have a higher binding affinity to LHRH receptors than naturally occurring LHRH and prolonged use of this range of drugs leads to desensitization of the gonadotrophin secreting cells in the pituitary gland and results in hypo-oestrogenism[1]. LHRH analogues are longer acting than naturally occurring LHRH since they are less susceptible to enzymatic degradation[2]. When an LHRH analogue is administered there is an initial stimulatory phase with a rise in the serum gonadotrophin levels and a rise in the resulting oestradiol level[3,4]. As the gonadal LH receptors reduce in number as the gonadotrophin levels rise, steroidogenesis will begin to decrease and the resultant state of hypogonadotrophic hypogonadism[5] which characterizes prolonged administration with LHRH agonists will continue until treatment ceases (Figure 1a and b).

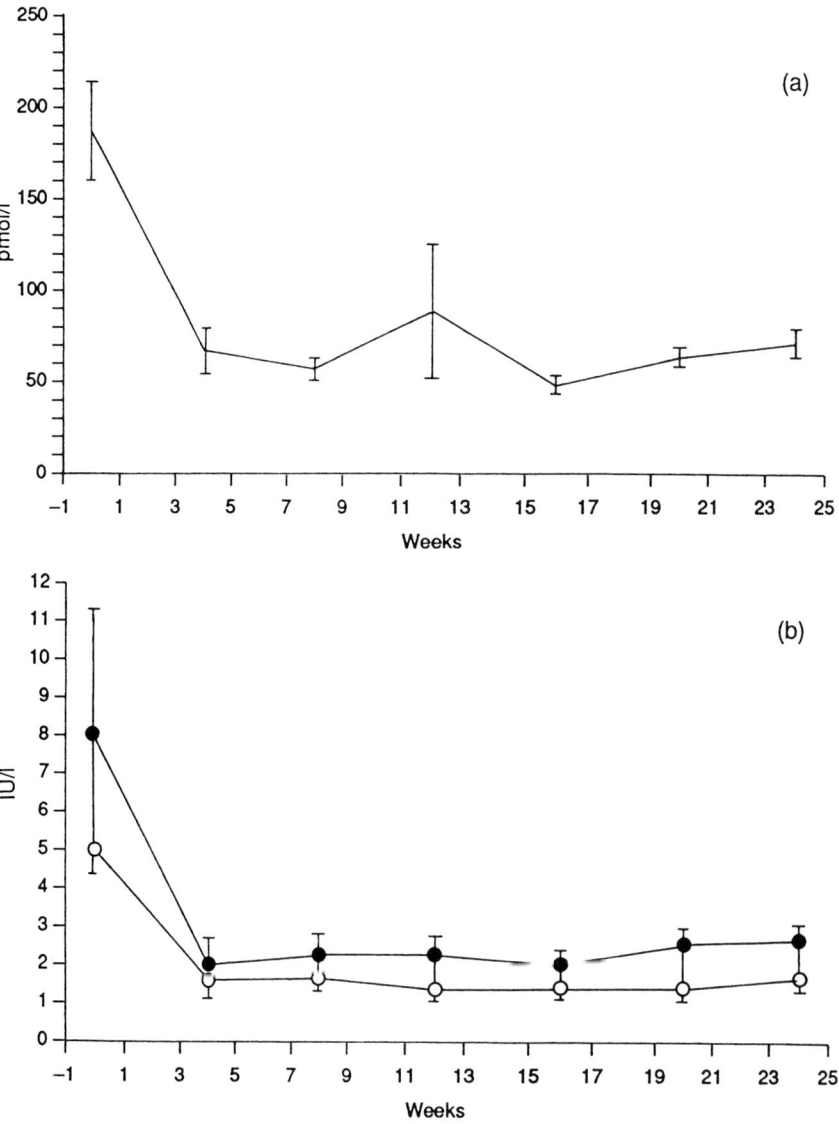

Figure 1 (a) Oestradiol levels (pmol/l) and (b) luteinizing hormone(●) and follicle stimulating hormone (○) (IU/l) during Zoladex therapy (3.6 mg Goserelin depot 4 weekly)

SIDE-EFFECTS OF LHRH ANALOGUES

Side-effects of LHRH analogues consist of those symptoms exhibited by women around the time of the menopause, namely hot flushes which vary in intensity and frequency with the individual, irritability, dryness of the vagina and loss of libido[6]. There are no significant serum lipid changes[7], but an unwanted side-effect of bone loss, which could potentially be significant if the treatment period is prolonged or repeated, may be a limiting factor in women undergoing LHRH analogue therapy for a benign condition such as menorrhagia[8,9].

At the same time that gonadotrophin and oestradiol levels are suppressed, patients commonly report vaginal bleeding when the LHRH analogue has been administered in the early follicular phase of the cycle. In 15 women treated for 6 months with the depot LHRH analogue goserelin (D-ser(tBu$_6$)AzGly$_{10}$LHRH) and where the mean cycle length was 28.2 days and the average duration of bleeding was 5.1 days, three had no vaginal bleeding whatsoever after administration of the first depot, four reported only spotting of blood, two complained of heavy bleeding and the remaining six reported only an average loss[10]. For the rest of the 6-month treatment period, none of the women reported any further vaginal bleeding, the menstrual cycle returning 8 to 12 weeks after administration of the last depot. This suggests that the depot's action lasts longer than the estimated 4 weeks in many women. At endometrial biopsy 4 weeks after the last depot had been inserted none of these women had sufficient endometrial tissue for histological examination.

LHRH ANALOGUE IN DYSFUNCTIONAL UTERINE BLEEDING

Animal data

In a study carried out by Fraser and Shaw on a colony of stump-tailed macaques[11], it was noted that several of these monkeys had excessive days of bleeding per menstrual cycle persisting for the 4-year study period. In five of these animals, the number of days of bleeding per month ranged from a mean of 7.5 to 15.4 days compared with a mean of 2.9 days in the remaining nine monkeys in the colony who had regular menses.

Pretreatment data on the five monkeys with abnormal bleeding indicated that the majority of cycles were normal ovulatory cycles in two, anovulatory in two and variable in the fifth. Beginning on day 1 of the cycle, two monkeys received 50 µg of the LHRH agonist buserelin (D-ser(tBu$_6$)desGly$_{10}$LHRH) daily by subcutaneous injection for 5 weeks and then the dose was reduced to 10 µg daily for the rest of the 6-month treatment period. The remaining three monkeys received 10 µg daily throughout the treatment period, one having the dose increased to 50 µg daily when improvement had not been achieved after 4 months of therapy.

During the first treatment cycle, all the monkeys bled for their usual duration. The two monkeys that received the initial 50 µg dose stopped bleeding thoughout the rest of the treatment period even when the dose was decreased to 10 µg per day. Two of the three monkeys that received the lower dose bled consistently but for shorter periods than in the pretreatment cycles and in the fifth animal where the dose was increased to 50 µg daily no improvement was observed even though there was ovarian suppression on measuring urinary hormonal levels.

Endometrial histology on these monkeys having been proven to be normal pretreatment, it showed decreased endometrial activity with inactive endometrium or only minimal proliferative activity. The animal that failed to respond had a thickened myometrium and fibroids. This study using the animal model suggested that ovarian suppression by means of an LHRH agonist could have a significant role to play in disorders of menstruation although excessive loss due to fibroids may prove more difficult to control.

Human studies

In normal ovulatory women, a daily dose of LHRH agonist administered to suppress ovulation will cause amenorrhoea in about a third of the women treated, while the remainder tend towards a reduction in the number of days of bleeding albeit at irregular intervals[12-14].

These studies, together with the animal study of the stump-tailed macaque, stimulated investigation of the effects of an LHRH agonist on dysfunctional uterine bleeding in women. In an initial small group of women, Shaw and Fraser investigated four who had undergone dilation and curettage under anaesthesia to exclude pelvic pathology[15]. Three months after curettage, none reported any improvement in their symptoms and all were reported to have an excessive loss of greater than 80 ml per cycle on measuring their menstrual blood loss by the alkaline haematin dilution technique[16]. The LHRH agonist buserelin was administered intranasally commencing on the 4th day of the cycle in a single daily dose of 400 μg in one and in a dose of 200 μg three times a day in the other three women. Treatment continued for 12 weeks during which the objective blood loss was assessed and was continued for two cycles after cessation of therapy.

The blood loss findings are summarized in Table 1. Pretreatment losses ranged from 95 to 198 ml per month and had been reduced to between nil and 30 ml during the second and third treatment cycles. The number of days menstrual bleeding after the first treatment cycle was also reduced except in one subject. The timing of the bleeding tended to become unpredictable, however, even though it was painless.

The patient who received the single daily dose of buserelin whilst achieving a substantial decrease in the amount of vaginal bleeding, bled for more days than in the pretreatment cycles and the urinary ovarian steroid patterns suggested that her previously ovulatory cycles had become anovulatory during treatment. These findings suggest that a more consistent pattern of ovarian suppression can be achieved by increasing the daily dose of buserelin to 600 μg daily and administering it

Table 1 Objective menstrual blood loss in ml per cycle in women with menorrhagia receiving buserelin intranasally. (From Shaw and Fraser, 1984[15], with permission)

		Patients			
		1	*2*	*3*	*4*
Pretreatment	1	143	94	162	108
cycles	2	186	112	148	98
Treatment	1	41	90	24	22
cycles	2	32	25	18	0
	3	28	15	0	0
Post-treatment	1	94	63	45	65
cycles	2	hysterectomy	88	372	102

in a divided dosage regimen. On cessation of therapy, cycles returned rapidly, the first menses occurring between 16 and 27 days after stopping buserelin and these cycles were ovulatory from the pattern of ovarian steroid hormones. In each patient the amount of measured menstrual blood loss increased markedly compared with the loss during therapy, ranging from 48 to 92 ml by the first period after cessation of therapy to 94 to 372 ml with the second.

As a result of studies being carried out at the Royal Free Hospital involving the use of LHRH agonists in the treatment of various benign gynaecological conditions, it is felt that depot LHRH preparations administered by subcutaneous injection every 4 weeks induce a more profound and sustained state of hypogonadotrophic hypogonadism when compared with the intranasal preparations. A group of six women with dysfunctional uterine bleeding have been studied in an ongoing study. All had a measured blood loss of greater than 80 ml per cycle using the alkaline haematin dilution technique, and following exclusion of uterine pathology goserelin depot was administered in a dose of 3.6 mg monthly for 3 months, the first depot being administered in the early follicular phase of the cycle. Menstrual losses during treatment and for three spontaneous cycles after cessation of therapy were also measured (Figure 2). There was a reduction in the menstrual blood loss in the first treatment cycle, and by the second cycle, five of the six women had amenorrhoea, the sixth woman losing only 2 ml. There was no loss in any of the women during the third treatment cycle or the first post-treatment cycle. Menses returned spontaneously in all women 7 to 10 weeks after the last depot had been inserted, much longer than in the study using buserelin for a similar length of time. In common with the buserelin study, the menses returned to their pretreatment volume.

Whether administered intranasally or by depot injection, LHRH agonists seem only to offer temporary relief of symptoms while treatment continues. The duration of the treatment period will have to be limited by the unwanted side-effect of bone loss making this range of drugs unsuitable for long-term use in the conservative management of menorrhagia in spite of their efficacy. Their role may well lie in the temporary relief of symptoms while patients wait their turn on the waiting list for a definitive surgical procedure or to tide them over in the short-term until the menopause has occurred. Achieving amenorrhoea during therapy may serve to lessen the incidence of blood transfusion

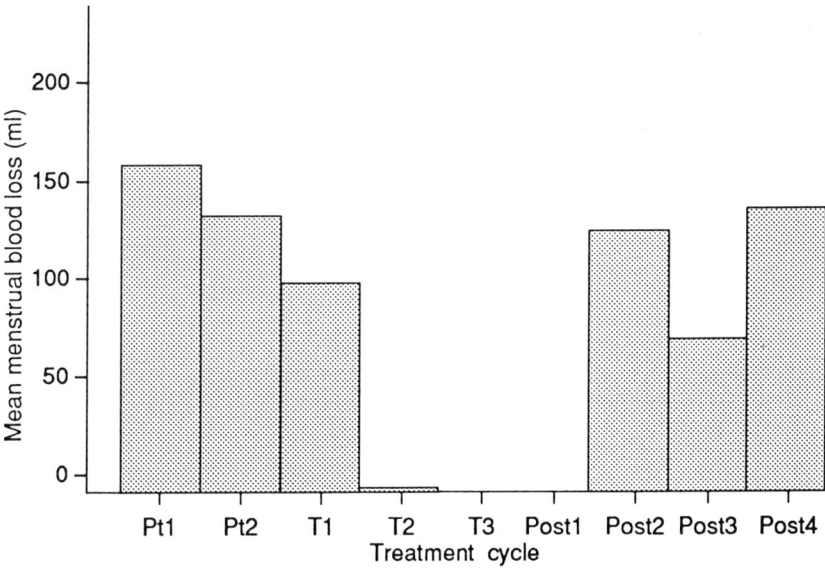

Figure 2   Mean menstrual blood loss (ml) before, during and after Zoladex depot

preoperatively and peroperatively since during LHRH agonist therapy, the haemoglobin concentrations of patients being treated will rise even where no iron therapy is administered (see below).

MENORRHAGIA IN ASSOCIATION WITH FIBROIDS

Menorrhagia is often one of the associated symptoms of fibroids and is probably the single most important symptom to the patient which precipitates presentation to the out-patient clinic and requires surgical treatment. Williams and Shaw at the Royal Free Hospital monitored the menstrual bleeding in a group of 11 women who underwent intranasal therapy with naferelin (D-(Nal$_2$)^6-LHRH) administered at a dose of 250 μg twice daily. These women had complained of excessive menstrual bleeding and all had uteri that were palpable per abdomen. The menstrual blood loss was assessed subjectively (Table 2). The pretreatment loss lasted a mean of 7.4 days and six of the 11 women had haemoglobin levels less than 11.4 g/dl. The therapy lasted 6 months. All 11 patients

Table 2 Number of days vaginal bleeding reported by patients undergoing therapy with naferelin 250 μg bd intranasally as treatment for fibroids or endometriosis

	Months of treatment					
Subjects	*1*	*2*	*3*	*4*	*5*	*6*
Fibroids						
A	8	1				
B	6					
C	18					
D	9					
E	11					
F	2	9				
G	8	11	8			
H	10	10	10	9	12	15
I	13	17	9	18	22	17
J	14	10	1	3	1	1
K	10	13	22	9	4	2
Endometriosis						
a	5					
b	13					
c	15					
d	14					
e	6					
f	5					
g	15					
h	8	4				
i	15	3		3		5
j	7	3	2			

experienced an increase in the duration of bleeding in the first treatment cycle but they all felt that the volume of bleeding was less than usual. Four patients experienced no further bleeding for the rest of the treatment period and three others reported only spotting of blood occasionally. The remaining four reported monthly losses throughout the treatment period , two stating that the loss was average for them and the other two reported excessive losses. At the end of the treatment period, all women had haemoglobin levels in excess of 12.5 g/dl without receiving any oral iron therapy. Where naferelin was used in the same dosage in women undergoing therapy for endometriosis, only four out of ten reported any vaginal bleeding during the treatment period after the initial treatment cycle and two had further scanty bleeding that did not require any sanitary protection. This suggests that where menorrhagia is associated with fibroids, the control of menstrual bleeding by an LHRH agonist is not as good as in the case of dysfunctional uterine bleeding. Similar results are being found in 20 women undergoing therapy for fibroids with the depot LHRH agonist goserelin at the Royal Free Hospital.

LHRH analogues have been widely reported as decreasing uterine volume and fibroid size during therapy[17-19]. Matta *et al.* report that using Doppler techniques the uterine artery blood supply to a fibroid uterus decreases with the use of the LHRH agonist buserelin which may in part account for the beneficial effect of LHRH agonist therapy in fibroids regarding shrinkage of the fibroids and lessening of the menstrual flow associated with fibroids[20].

After cessation of LHRH analogue therapy, fibroids are well known to regrow and therefore LHRH analogues are only of temporary benefit in the management of fibroid-associated menorrhagia. Matta and Shaw report that 6 months after cessation of therapy with buserelin fibroid volumes had returned to or exceeded pretreatment volumes[21]. Since the control of menorrhagia associated with fibroids is not 100% effective, coupled with the fact that the benefit of shrinkage lasts only while treatment continues, the LHRH analogues may be of benefit in the preoperative period to build up the patient's haemoglobin levels, and shrink the fibroids to facilitate surgery. It may also be expected that diminution of the uterine artery blood flow may facilitate surgery and possibly make myomectomy, in particular, a safer procedure.

CONCLUSIONS

LHRH analogues are well tolerated drugs that control dysfunctional uterine bleeding and to a lesser extent the excessive menses associated with fibroids. Their effect only lasts while therapy continues and prolonged treatment alone is prohibited by the unwanted side-effect of bone loss although combination therapy regimen may overcome this. Their role in the management of menorrhagia therefore seems to be in the short-term while the patient awaits surgery or a spontaneous menopause, and in common with all other medical treatments for this condition, is not curative.

REFERENCES

1. Clayton, R.N. (1982). Gonadotrophin-releasing hormone modulation of its own pituitary receptors: evidence for biphasic regulation. *Endocrinology*, **111**, 152–61
2. Horsthemke, B., Knitsatschek, H., Rivier, J., Sandow, J. and Bauer, K. (1981). Degradation of luteinising hormone-releasing hormone and its analogs by adenohypophyseal peptidases. *Biochem. Biophys. Res. Commun.*, **100**, 753
3. Lemay, A., Maheux, R., Faure, N., Jean, C. and Fazekas, A. (1984). Reversible hypogonadism induced by a luteinising hormone-releasing hormone (LHRH) agonist (buserelin) as a new therapeutic approach for endometriosis. *Fertil. Steril.*, **41**, 863–71
4. Matta, W., Shaw, R. and Burford, G. (1988). Endocrinologic and clinical evaluation following a single administration of a gonadotropin-releasing hormone agonist (Zoladex) in depot formulation to premenopausal women. *Fertil. Steril.*, **49**, 163–5
5. Meldrum, D., Chang, R., Lu, J., Vale, W., Rivier, J. and Judd, H. (1982). Medical oophorectomy using a long-acting GnRH agonist – a possible new approach to the treatment of endometriosis. *J. Clin. Endocrinol. Metab.*, **54**, 1081–3
6. Matta, W. and Shaw, R. (1986). A comparative study between buserelin and danazol in the treatment of endometriosis. *Br. J. Clin. Pract.*, Suppl., **48**, 64–8
7. Crook, D., Gardner, R., Nolan, J., Stevenson, J. and Shaw, R. (1988). Zoladex v Danazol in endometriosis: effects on plasma lipids, lipoproteins and apolipoproteins. *Presented at the International Symposium on Endocrine Therapy*, Monaco, 19–21 November 1988
8. Stevenson, J., Lees, B., Gardner, R. and Shaw, R. (1989). Prolonged effects of an LHRH agonist, goserelin, on the skeleton. *Presented at the Silver Jubilee British Congress of Obstetrics and Gynaecology*, London, 4–7 July 1989
9. Matta, W., Shaw, R., Hesp, R. and Evans, R. (1988). Reversible trabecular bone density loss following induced hypo-oestrogenism with the LHRH analogue buserelin in premonopausal women. *Clin. Endocrinol.*, **29**, 45–51
10. Gardner, R. and Shaw, R. (1988). Patterns of hot flushes and vaginal bleeding in patients being treated with Zoladex Depot (goserelin, ICI 118,630) for endometriosis. *Presented at the International Symposium on GnRH analogues in Cancer and Human Reproduction*, Geneva, Switzerland, 18–21 February 1988
11. Fraser, H. and Shaw, R. (1984). Effects of chronic luteinising hormone-

158

releasing hormone agonist treatment in dysfunctional uterine bleeding in the stump-tailed macaque. *Acta Endocrinol.*, **106**, 381–6

12. Bergquist, C., Nillius, S. and Wide, L. (1982). Long term intranasal luteinising hormone-releasing hormone agonist treatment for contraception in women. *Fertil. Steril.*, **38**, 190–3

13. Schmidt-Gollwitzer, M., Hardt, W., Schmidt-Gollwitzer, K., Vonder Ohne, M. and Nevinny-Stickel, J. (1981). Influence of the LH-RH analogue buserelin on cyclic ovarian function and on endometrium. A new approach to fertility control? *Contraception*, **23**, 187–95

14. Bergquist, C., Nillius, S., Wide, L. and Lingren, A. (1981). Endometrial patterns in women on chronic luteinising hormone-releasing hormone agonist treatment for contraception. *Fertil. Steril.*, **36**, 339–42

15. Shaw, R. and Fraser, H. (1984). Use of a superactive luteinising hormone-releasing hormone agonist in the treatment of menorrhagia. *Br. J. Obstet. Gynaecol.*, **91**, 913–16

16. Hallberg, L. and Nilsson, L. (1964). Determination of menstrual blood loss. *Scand. J. Clin. Lab. Invest.*, **16**, 244–8

17. West, C., Lumsden, M.A., Lawson, S., Williamson, J. and Baird, D. (1987). Shrinkage of uterine fibroids during therapy with goserelin (Zoladex) a luteinising hormone-releasing hormone agonist administered as a monthly subcutaneous depot. *Fertil. Steril.*, **48**, 45–51

18. Perl, V., Marquez, J., Schally, A., Comaru-Schally, A., Leal, G., Zacharias, S. and Gomez-Lira, C. (1987). Treatment of leiomyomata uteri with D-Trp6-luteinising hormone releasing hormone. *Fertil. Steril.*, **48**, 383–9

19. Maheux, R., Lemay, A. and Merat, P. (1987). Use of intranasal luteinising hormone-releasing hormone agonist in uterine leimyomatas. *Fertil. Steril.*, **47**, 229–33

20. Matta, W.H.M., Stabile, I., Shaw, R. and Campbell, S. (1988). Doppler assessment of uterine blood flow changes in patients with fibroids receiving the gonadotropin-releasing hormone agonist buserelin. *Fertil. Steril.*, **49**, 1083–5

21. Matta, W.H.M., Shaw, R.W. and Nye, M. (1989). Long-term follow-up of patients with uterine fibroids after treatment with the LHRH agonist buserelin. *Br. J. Obstet. Gynaecol.*, **96**, 200–6

DISCUSSION

Dr M.A. Lumsden We found – looking at the effect of Zoladex combined with tamoxifen – that when we started treatment at the onset of the menses, there was immediate cessation of the menses and there was no further bleeding while treatment was carried on. Subsequently we have used it in one or two cases with acute admission for torrential bleeding with enormous success.

Secondly, we have treated now quite a large number of women with fibroids with Zoladex and we find it extremely effective at inducing amenorrhoea. Very few women have dysfunctional bleeding, and those that do, it really has not been a nuisance.

Prof. R.W. Shaw Presumably the rationale for the administration of an analogue in someone with acute severe haemorrhage is that in fact an oestrogen surge is induced. It is rather like giving a bolus of Premarin, because they get an agonistic increase in oestrogen, which may be the controlling agent for the acute haemorrhage.

Mr E. Versi It strikes me that one of the problems with Zoladex is the worries about the bone loss in the long term. But there are agents that are being developed that may well spare bone. Vaginal dryness was mentioned. I was wondering if anybody had had any experience of using oestriol cream along with Zoladex. It will not have a significant effect on the uterus and it is unlikely to cause any bleeding.

Dr R. Gardner No. We certainly have not used any oestrogen-containing creams in the vagina.

But I reported those as recognized side-effects, and I think out of about 130 women that I have treated with Zoladex, only two have complained of severe vaginal dryness.

Index

age
  and menorrhagia 41
  and tolerance of menorrhagia 60
alkaline haematin, method of blood
  loss measurement 13
anaemia
  iron deficiency 13, 60, 85
angiogenesis 4
anovulatory dysfunctional uterine
  bleeding, diagnosis of 139
antifibrinolytic agents 91
arachidonic acid 5
  synthesis 45
Asherman syndrome 97

breakthrough bleeding 1, 92, 134,
  142
  progesterone as a cause 2
buserelin 153, 157

calcium
  and phospholipase activity 45
  effect on prostaglandin synthesis 5
carcinoma
  and progestogen therapy 143
  risks of after resection 116
colony-stimulating factor 1, 6
contraception
  intrauterine 25, 60, 144
  oral 1, 143
corpus luteum,
  role in menstruation 1

cystic glandular hyperplasia 128, 142

danazol 61, 89, 120, 128–136, 148
definitions of menorrhagia 66, 139
depot medroxyprogesterone
  acetate 143
diclofenac 117
dysmenorrhoea
  and menorrhagia 119
  response to mefenamic acid 122

ectopic pregnancy rate with
  intrauterine devices 148
endometrial ablation
  by hysteroscopy 97
  early methods 97
endometrial diathermy/resection 99
endometrium
  lysosomal content 3
  proliferation of 6
  regeneration of 4, 6
  response to danazol 129
  response to progestogens 140
  vasculature of 26
epidermal growth factor 6
  synergism with oestradiol 10

fibrin, in menstrual blood 29
fibrinogen breakdown products in
  menorrhagia 32
fibrinolysis and menorrhagia 31
fibrinolytic activity 25

fibroids
  and menorrhagia 49, 155
  as a reason for hysterectomy 87

goserelin 157
growth factors, effect on
  phospholipases 58

haemostasis 19
  morphology of 27
  role in menstruation 3
history of blood loss,
  importance of 59
hormone replacement therapy 1, 116
hysterectomy
  as a cure for menstrual disorders 13
  as a treatment for menorrhagia 84
  cost of 85
  incidence of 87
hysteroscopy, as a treatment for
  menorrhagia 92

ibuprofen 117
  and menstrual blood loss
  reduction 18
intrauterine surgery, risks of 109
intravenous sedation, use in
  resections 105
iron deficiency anaemia 13, 60, 85
ischaemia, distal 3

lasers
  use in endometrial ablation 98
  use in endometrial resection 92
leukotriene synthesis 15
leukotrienes 13
LHRH agonists 91
LHRH analogues
  mode of action 149
  side-effects of 151
lysosomes, role in menstruation 3

medical treatment
  cost of 91
  of menorrhagia 88
medroxyprogesterone acetate 142,
  143, 147
mefenamic acid 89, 117, 120, 148
  and menstrual blood loss
  reduction 18
menorrhagia
  and dysmenorrhoea 119
  and fibroids 49, 155
  cost of therapy with danazol 136
  cost to health service 85
  definitions of 60, 66, 139
  medical treatment of 88
  psychological aspects of 67
  response to danazol 129
  therapy with LHRH
  analogues 151–157
  treatment by endometrial
  ablation 97
  treatment by hysterectomy 84
  treatment by hysteroscopy 92
  treatment with progestogens 140
menstrual blood loss
  and parity 24
  duration of 64, 122
  evaluation of 59
  heaviness of 59
  history of 59
  measurement by catheter 120, 125
  measurement by haemoglobin
  determination 70, 72
  measurement by iron
  determination 70, 72
  measurement by pictorial blood loss
  assessment chart 74–78
  measurement by radioisotope
  methods 70, 71
  measurement by weight
  estimates 70

objective measurement 13
quantification 69
reduction by prostaglandin synthesis
  inhibitors 4
regulating factors 1
skewed distribution of 13
subjective assessment of 61
menstrual coagulation 31
menstrual fluid
composition of 3, 81
menstruation
anovulatory cycles 2
endocrine control of 1
regular ovulatory cycles 2
role of prostaglandins in 4
theories of mechanism 2
mental disturbance, and menstrual
  blood loss 60
myometrium, phospholipase
activity of 50

naferelin 156
naproxen 117
norethisterone 89, 134, 142, 147

oestradiol 6
role in menstruation 1
synergism with epidermal growth
  factor 10
oestrogen, effect on epidermal growth
  factor 9
osteoporosis 92, 116, 154

pad counting 62
parity
and menorrhagia 41
and menstrual blood loss 24
phospholipase A_2 5
activity 45
in menorrhagia 44
phospholipase, C 5, 17

activity 53
pictorial blood loss assessment
  chart 74–78
plasminogen activator in
  menorrhagia 33
platelet fibrin plug formation 3
platelets, in menstrual blood 29
polycystic ovary syndrome
and phospholipase A_2 activity 51
phospholipase levels in 44
progesterone, role in menstruation 1
progesterone as a cause of
  breakthrough bleeding 2
progestogens
administration methods 141
effect on endometrium 141
use in menorrhagia 140
prostacyclin
in menorrhagia 17
ratio to thromboxane in
  menorrhagia 5
prostaglandin $F_{2\alpha}$ 5
prostaglandin production 10
prostaglandin synthetase 5
prostaglandin synthetase inhibitors,
  use in menorrhagia
  therapy 117–123
prostaglandins
abnormal levels in menorrhagia 13
and endometrial function 5
and epidermal growth factor 11
biosynthetic pathways 16
isolation of 14
production in menorrhagia 16–18
role in dysfunctional uterine
  bleeding 15
role in menstruation 4, 43
structure of 14
synthesis 5
psychological aspects of
  menorrhagia 67

regeneration, role in menstruation 4
risks of intrauterine surgery 109

side-effects
    of danazol 135, 138
    of LHRH analogues 151
    of medical therapies 89
    of mefenamic acid 122
    of progestogens 143
    of prostaglandin synthetase
      inhibitors 119
society
    role of women in 1, 59
steroid, peripheral levels and
    menstruation 2
subjective assessment of menstrual
    blood loss 61

tamoxifen 159
tampon counting 62
thrombocytopenia 6

thromboxane, ratio to prostacyclin in
    menorrhagia 5
transcervical resection of the
    endometrium 100–112
transforming growth factors 6

ultrastructural studies of menstrual
    platelets 20
uterine size, reduction after danazol
    therapy 131
uterine volume and menstrual blood
    loss 69

vascular changes, role in
    menstruation 2
von Willebrand disease 6

withdrawal bleeding 1

Zoladex 159